DSM-5-TR Insanely Simplified

DSM-5-TR INSANELY SIMPLIFIED

Unlocking the Spectrums within DSM-5-TR and ICD 10

Steven Buser, MD
&
Leonard Cruz, MD

Illustrations by Luke Sloan

CHIRON PUBLICATIONS • ASHEVILLE, NORTH CAROLINA

© 2022 by Chiron Publications. All rights reserved. No part of this publication may be reproduced, stored in a retrieval system, or transmitted, in any form by any means, electronic, mechanical, photocopying, recording, or otherwise, without the prior written permission of the publisher, Chiron Publications, PO Box 19690, Asheville, NC 28815
www.ChironPublicatons.com

Cover design by Cornelia G. Murariu & Danijela Mijailovic
Interior by Danijela Mijailovic
Printed in the United States of America

DSM-5-TR is a registered trademark of the American Psychiatric Association. The APA did not participate in the preparation of this book.

ISBN 978-1-68503-044-5 paperback
ISBN 978-1-68503-045-2 hardcover
ISBN 978-1-68503-046-9 electronic
978-1-68503-047-6 limited edition paperback

Library of Congress Cataloging-in-Publication Data

Names: Buser, Steven, 1963- author. | Cruz, Leonard, 1957- author.
Title: DSM-5-TR insanely simplified : unlocking the spectrums within DSM-5-TR and ICD 10 / Steven Buser, MD & Leonard Cruz, MD ; illustrations by Luke Sloan.
Description: Asheville, North Carolina : Chiron Publications, [2022] | Includes bibliographical references and index. | Summary: "The publication of the Diagnostic and Statistical Manual Version 5 (DSM-5, 2013) and the more recent Diagnostic and Statistical Manual Version 5 - Text Revision edition (DSM-5-TR, 2022), together ushered in a major change to the field of mental health diagnosis. DSM-5-TR Insanely Simplified provides a summary of key concepts of the new diagnostic schema introduced in DSM-5 as well as the updated DSM-5-TR. It utilizes a variety of techniques to help clinicians master the new spectrum approach to diagnosis and its complex criteria. Cartoons, mnemonic devices, and summary tables allow clinicians and students to quickly grasp and retain broad concepts and subtle nuances related to psychiatric diagnosis. DSM-5-TR Insanely Simplified fosters quick mastery of the most important concepts introduced in DSM-5 and continued in DSM-5-TR, while offering an entirely new way of looking at mental health along a continuum. This new approach goes beyond simply "labeling" clients with various diagnoses, but rather places them along spectrums that range from normal to problematic symptoms. Mental health professionals and laypeople will appreciate the synthesis of deep psychology and modern approaches to the diagnosis of mental illness"-- Provided by publisher.
Identifiers: LCCN 2022028585 (print) | LCCN 2022028586 (ebook) | ISBN 9781685030445 (paperback) | ISBN 9781685030452 (hardcover) | ISBN 9781685030476 (limited edition paperback) | ISBN 9781685030469 (ebook)
Subjects: LCSH: Diagnostic and statistical manual of mental disorders. 5th ed. | International statistical classification of diseases and related health problems. 10th revision. | Mental illness--Classification--Handbooks, manuals, etc. | Mental illness--Diagnosis--Handbooks, manuals, etc.
Classification: LCC RC455.2.C4 B874 2022 (print) | LCC RC455.2.C4 (ebook) | DDC 616.89/075--dc23/eng/20220713
LC record available at https://lccn.loc.gov/2022028585
LC ebook record available at https://lccn.loc.gov/2022028586

*To our wives, Megan and Vicky, and our children,
Brian, Emily, Saila, and Sarah
And all their amazing love and inspiration
that fuel our life's work.*

CONTENTS

DSM-5-TR Summary Pages	ix

Section I: Overview — 1
1. Introduction — 3
2. History of the DSM — 9
3. What is new in DSM-5-TR — 15
4. What was new in DSM-5 — 19
5. The 8 Primary Psychiatric Spectrums of Mental Illness — 29

Section II: The 8 Primary Spectrums of Psychiatry — 37
6. The Depression Spectrum: Shallowness vs. Despair — 39
7. The Mania Spectrum: Boring vs. Bipolar — 47
8. The Anxiety Spectrum: Carelessness vs. Anxiousness — 53
9. The Psychosis Spectrum: Visionless vs. Psychotic — 59
10. The Focus Spectrum: Attention Deficit Disorder vs. Obsessive Compulsive Disorders — 65
11. The Substance Abuse Spectrum: Ascetic vs. Addicted — 73
12. The Autism Spectrum: Codependent vs. Autistic — 81
13. The Personality Spectrum: Neurotic vs. Obnoxious — 87

Section III: The Secondary Areas of Diagnosis — 93
14. The Specialty Areas (Trauma, Neurodevelopmental, Neurocognitive, Behavioral, Dissociative, Somatic, Eating, Elimination, Sleep, Sexual, Gender, Paraphilia) — 95

Section IV: Conclusions — **101**
15. The Harmony of the Lotus Flower — 103
16. Carl Jung and his Relationship to DSM-5-TR — 105

Appendix: On ICD-10 and the DSM-5-TR — **107**

Endnotes — 109

Index — 113

DSM-5-TR SUMMARY PAGES

WARNING! The descriptions of DSM-5-TR disorders that follow are in a highly simplified and summarized form. They are meant to give a quick overview and a reminder of each disorder. They do not, however, include all of the full diagnostic criteria found in the complete DSM-5-TR text. The DSM-5-TR is available as a separate text. Please do not use this book to formally reach a diagnosis, but rather as a quick reference and memory tool.

All codes employed in this book pertain to the DSM-5-TR as well as ICD-10. Older ICD-9 codes are no longer relevant.

DEPRESSIVE DISORDERS

Major Depressive Disorder
- 5 "SIG E CAPSS" symptoms for at least 2 weeks [**S**adness, **I**nterest loss, **G**uilt or worthlessness, **E**nergy loss, **C**oncentration loss, **A**ppetite change, **P**sychomotor agitation or retardation, **S**leep change, **S**uicidal thoughts]

F32.x   **Major Depressive Disorder, single episode**
F32.0-mild;   F32.1-mod.; F32.2 – severe; F32.3 - psychotic; F32.4-partial remission; F32.5-full remission, F32.9-unspecified

F33.x   **Major Depressive Disorder, recurrent**
F33.0-mild; F33.1-mod.; F33.2 – severe; F33.3 - psychotic; F33.41-partial remission; F33.42-full rem. F33.9-unspecified

F34.1 Persistent Depressive Disorder (Dysthymia)
- Sad most days for 2 years
- 2 or more of: sleep change, hopelessness, appetite change, low self-esteem, concentration loss
- Never 2 months symptom free in first 2 years
- Significant distress or impairment

F43.8 Prolonged Grief Disorder
- Death of a loved one, 1 year ago or more (6 months for children)
- Near constant intense yearning or preoccupation with memories of deceased
- Significant distress
- 3 or more symptoms most days of: loneliness, meaninglessness, emotional numbness, identity disruption, denial of their death, avoiding reminders, intense emotional pain, or can't resume with activities & friends

F32.81 Premenstrual Dysphoric Disorder
- Symptoms present one week prior to menses (period)
- At least 1 of the following 4 is present: mood swings, irritability/anger, sadness, anxiety/tension
- At least 5 total: mood swings, irritability/anger, sadness, anxiety/ tension, loss of interest, poor concentration, fatigue, appetite change, sleep change, overwhelmed, physical symptoms (breast tenderness, bloating, pain, weight gain)
- Significant distress or impairment

F34.81 Disruptive Mood Dysregulation Disorder
- Severe recurrent temper outbursts (verbal or physical)
- Out of proportion to context
- 3 or more per week; persists more than a year; began as child (6-18)
- Persistent irritability
- (not better explained by mania, depression, autism, substance abuse, etc)

F32.A Unspecified Mood Disorder

BIPOLAR DISORDERS

F31.9 Bipolar I Disorder
- Euphoric or irritable mood and increased energy or activity for 1 week
- 3 out of 7: grandiose, decreased sleep, talkative, racing thoughts, distractibility, increased goal-directed activity, impulsive
- Social or work impairment

F31.81 Bipolar II Disorder
- At least 1 Hypomanic episode and at least 1 Major Depressive episode
- No full Manic episodes

Hypomanic Episode:
- Same as Bipolar I Manic episode except: at least 4 days duration (instead of 7)
- And **NO marked impairment** in social or occupational functioning

F34.0 Cyclothymic Disorder
- Numerous hypomania and depression symptoms for most of the time for 2 years
- Never reaches full diagnosis for either hypomanic, manic or depressive episodes
- Not without symptoms for 2 months in 1st 2 years.
- Clinically significant distress or impairment

May Add Specifiers:
- with Anxious Distress
- with Mixed Features (mania and depression)
- with Rapid Cycling (for Bipolar I and II: > 4 episodes per year)
- with Melancholic Features (loss of pleasure, lack of reactivity, despair, worse in a.m., early morning awakening)
- with Atypical Features (weight gain, increased sleep, leaden paralysis, interpersonal rejection sensitivity, mood reactivity)
- with Psychotic Features
- with Catatonia
- with Peripartum Onset
- with Seasonal Pattern

PSYCHOTIC DISORDERS

F20.9 Schizophrenia
- Must have 1 positive symptom (hallucinations, delusions, or disorganized speech) for 1 month
- 2 of the following: hallucinations, delusions, disorganized speech, disorganized behavior, or negative symptoms (low emotion, low motivation)
- Prior or residual poor functioning for at least 6 months
- Social or work impairment

F20.81 Schizophreniform Disorder
- Schizophrenic symptoms between 1-6 months duration

F25.1 Schizoaffective Disorder, Depressive type
- Schizophrenic symptoms and Depression symptoms present most of the time.
- At least 2 weeks of delusions or hallucinations without Depression symptoms
- Must have Depression symptoms for the majority of time

F25.0 Schizoaffective Disorder, Bipolar type
- Schizophrenic symptoms and Bipolar I symptoms present most of the time
- At least 2 weeks of delusions or hallucinations without Bipolar symptoms
- Must have Bipolar symptoms for the majority of time

F23 Brief Psychotic Disorder
- Schizophrenic symptoms for less than 1 month
- Full return to premorbid level
  - with marked stressors
  - without marked stressors
  - with postpartum onset
  - with Catatonia

F22 Delusional Disorder
- Moderate delusions at least 1 month, not Schizophrenic level
- Otherwise good functioning; no bizarre behavior
  - Erotomanic type
  - Grandiose type
  - Jealous type
  - Somatic type
  - Mixed type
  - Unspecified type
  - Persecutory type

ANXIETY DISORDERS

F41.0 Panic Disorder
- Recurrent, abrupt, unexpected intense fear or discomfort
- Persistent worry of additional attacks for 1 month
- 4 out of 13 symptoms: (palpitations, sweating, trembling, shortness of breath, choking, chest pain, nausea, dizziness, derealization, fear of "going crazy", fear of dying, numbness/tingling, hot/cold flashes)
- "Panic Attack" can also be a specifier for other diagnoses (i.e. "PTSD with Panic Attacks")

F41.1 Generalized Anxiety Disorder
- Excessive worry most days for 6 months
- 3 out of 6: (restless, fatigue, decreased concentration, irritability, tense, insomnia)
- Interferes with work / social functioning

F40.10 Social Anxiety Disorder
- Formerly "Social Phobia"
- Persistent fear of social interaction or performance
- Interferes with work / social functioning

F40.00 Agoraphobia
- Intense fear of 2 or more of the following: public transportation, open spaces (markets, bridges), enclosed spaced (theaters, shops), crowds, being away from home
- Avoids these areas
- Greater than 6 months; interferes with work or social functioning

F93.0 Separation Anxiety Disorder
- Excessive anxiety over separation from home or parents

F94.0 Selective Mutism
Mute in some settings but not others; lasts at least 1 month

Specific Phobias
- Intense unreasonable fear
- Interferes with work / social functioning
- F40.218 - Animal fear (insects, snakes, dogs, etc)
- F40.228 - Natural environment (heights, thunderstorms, etc)
- F40.230 - Blood
- F40.231 - Needle injections
- F40.232 - Other medical fears
- F40.233 - Fear of injury
- F40.248 - Situational (elevators, planes, tight spaces)
- F40.298 - Other

OBSESSIVE-COMPULSIVE DISORDERS

F42.2 Obsessive-Compulsive Disorder
- Obsessions: persistent intrusive, unwanted, inappropriate mostly non-psychotic thoughts
- Compulsions: repetitive behaviors driven to perform in response to obsessions intended to reduce distress & anxiety
- Patient perceives as excessive / unreasonable
- Marked distress / interference; time consuming (> 1 hour / day)

Add Specifier:
- with good or fair insight
- with poor insight
- with absent insight/delusional beliefs

F63.3 Trichotillomania
- Recurrent hair pulling and hair loss
- Failed attempts to stop hair pulling
- Marked distress or impairment

F42.3 Hoarding Disorder
- Can't discard possessions regardless of value
- Possessions accumulate, cluttering living space
- Marked distress or impairment

F42.4 Excoriation (Skin-Picking) Disorder
- Persistent skin picking causing lesions or infections
- Failed attempts to stop skin picking
- Not related to substance use (cocaine, methamphetamine, etc.)
- Marked distress or impairment

F45.22 Body Dysmorphic Disorder
- Preoccupation with imagined defect in physical appearance
- Repetitive checking, grooming, picking, comparing, or reassurance seeking
- Work / social impairment

SUBSTANCE ABUSE DISORDERS

Alcohol Use Disorder
F10.10 MILD = 2-3 symptoms
F10.20 MOD = 4-5 symptoms
F10.20 SEV = 6 or more symptoms

Addiction Symptom List:
- Uses more than intended
- Failed attempts to cut back
- Excessive time spent obtaining, using, or recovering from substance
- Cravings for substance
- Substance use leads to problems at work, school or home
- Work, social, or recreational activities are given up due to substance use
- Uses in dangerous situations
- Persistent use despite awareness of problem
- Tolerance (needs more substance for same effect)
- Withdrawals
- Use despite negative effects

	Mild:	Mod/Sev:	
Opioid Use Disorder	F11.10	F11.20	[or Intoxication/Withdrawal]
Alcohol Use Disorder	F10.10	F10.20	[or Intoxication/Withdrawal]
Stimulant Use Disorder	F15.10	F15.20	[or Intoxication/Withdrawal]
Sedative Use Disorder	F13.10	F13.20	[or Intoxication/Withdrawal]
Cannabis Use Disorder	F12.10	F12.20	[or Intoxication/Withdrawal]
Tobacco Use Disorder	Z72.0	F17.200	[or Withdrawal]
Hallucinogen Use Disorder	F16.10	F16.20	[or Intoxication]
Inhalant Use Disorder	F18.10	F18.20	[or Intoxication]
Other (Unknown) Substance Use Disorder	F19.10	F19.20	

F63.0 Gambling Disorder
- Continued problematic gambling despite distress or impairment
- 4 of the following: increasing amounts of money gambled, irritable when cuts back on gambling, failed attempts to cut back, preoccupied with gambling, gambles to feel better, "chases their losses" (gambles later to make their money back), lies about gambling, relationship / work / or school problems, others give them money to help desperate need caused by losses

NEURODEVELOPMENTAL DISORDERS

Attention-Deficit / Hyperactivity Disorder (ADHD)
- Persistent **inattention** or **hyperactivity** interfering with functioning for 6 months, beginning before age of 12
- **Inattention** - 6 or more of the following: inattention to details, difficulty sustaining attention, doesn't listen well, poor follow through on tasks, poor organization, avoids homework or large projects, often loses things, distractible, forgetful
- **Hyperactivity** - 6 or more of the following: fidgets or squirms, leaves seat often, runs around inappropriately, can't play quietly, driven, always moving, overly talkative, blurts out answers, difficulty waiting or taking turns, interrupts frequently

F90.2 ADHD, Combined
F90.0 ADHD, Inattentive
F90.1 ADHD, Hyperactive / Impulsive

F84.0 Autism Spectrum Disorder:
Problems with social communication and social interaction Repetitive behaviors; 2 of the following:
- Repetitive actions or speech
- Insistence on sameness
- Restricted fixated interests
- Increased or decreased sensitivity to sensory stimulation

3 Levels:
Level 1 - requiring support
Level 2 - requiring substantial support
Level 3 - requiring very substantial support

Intellectual Disability:
F70 - Mild
F71 - Moderate
F72 - Severe
F73 - Profound
- Decreased intellectual functioning
- Decreased developmental and social functioning
- Begins in childhood

Communication Disorders:
F80.2 Language Disorder - difficulty using language
F80.0 Speech Sound Disorder - difficulty speaking
F80.81 Childhood Onset Fluency Disorder - stuttering issues
F80.82 Social (Pragmatic) Communication Disorder - speaking difficulties in social context

Specific Learning Disorders:
F81.0 - Reading
F81.81 - Writing
F81.2 - Mathematics

TRAUMA AND STRESS DISORDERS

F43.10 Post Traumatic Stress Disorder (PTSD)
- Severe Trauma - experienced trauma, witnessed trauma, or learned about violent trauma to loved one
- Intrusive memories, nightmares, flashbacks
- Avoidance - (avoid memories, thoughts, feelings, reminders)
- Negative thoughts & feelings: amnesia to the event, exaggerated negative beliefs, self (or other) blame, persistent fear / anger/ horror / shame, low interest in activities, feeling detached, feeling numb
- Hyperarousal (insomnia, poor concentration, emotional lability, hypervigilance, exaggerated startle, reckless or self-destructive behavior)
- Symptoms present for 1 month and work / social impairment

Note if Preschool Subtype (under 6 years of age)

F43.0 Acute Stress Disorder
- PTSD, but less than one month since trauma

F43.2x Adjustment Disorders
- Stressor leading to excessive distress or work / social impairment
- Symptoms do not last greater than 6 months after resolution of stress
- Specify stress as acute or chronic (greater than 6 months)

F43.21 Adjustment Disorder with depressed mood
F43.22 Adjustment Disorder with anxiety
F43.23 Adjustment Disorder with mixed anxiety and depressed mood
F43.24 Adjustment Disorder with disturbance of conduct
F43.25 Adjustment Disorder with mixed disturbance of emotions and conduct

F94.1 Reactive Attachment Disorder
- Poor caregiving at early age (neglected, deprived, too numerous care-givers, or orphanage)
- Emotionally withdrawn behavior towards care-givers (doesn't seek or respond to comfort)
- Socially and emotionally unresponsive, inappropriately irritable / sad / or fearful

F94.2 Disinhibited Social Engagement Disorder
- Poor care-giving at early age (neglected, deprived, too numerous care-givers, or orphanage)
- Child inappropriately approaches or is overly familiar with unknown adult

MOTOR DISORDERS

F95.2 Tourette's Disorder
- Multiple motor tics + 1 vocal tic
- Persistent for 1 year
- Marked distress or impairment
- Onset before 18 years old

F95.0 Provisional Tic Disorder
- Tics, 4 weeks to 1 year
- Marked distress or impairment
- Onset before 18 years old

F95.1 Persistent Motor or Vocal Tic Disorder
- Motor only or vocal only tics
- Persistent for 1 year
- Marked distress or impairment
- Onset before 18 years old

F98.4 Stereotypic movement Disorder
- Repetitive purposeless movement (head banging, rocking, biting, picking, hitting, etc.)
- Interferes with functioning or self-injurious

F82 Developmental Coordination Disorder
- Coordination impairment, clumsy, slow, inaccurate
- Marked distress / interference

DISSOCIATIVE DISORDERS

F44.81 Dissociative Identity Disorder (Multiple Personality)
- 2 or more distinct personalities recurrently take control
- Compartmentalization of information
- Marked distress or impairment

F48.1 Depersonalization / Derealization Disorder
- Recurrent subjective detachment (as if an "outside observer" or in a dream)
- Intact reality testing (not psychotic)
- Marked distress or impairment

F44.0 Dissociative Amnesia
- Trauma leading to inability to remember personal information
- Marked distress or impairment
- Specify if it includes **Dissociative Fugue (travel) F44.1**

EATING DISORDERS

F50.0x Anorexia Nervosa
- Restriction of food intake and refusal to maintain minimally healthy weight
- Strong fear of gaining weight or being "fat"
- Disturbance in body image (usually perceiving self as much heavier)
- Mild: BMI above 17, Moderate: BMI 16-16.99, Severe: BMI 15 - 15.99, Extreme: BMI <15
  F50.01 Restricting Type - no binge eating or purging (purely uses fasting and exercising)
  F50.02 Binge / Purge type - some binges or purging (vomiting, laxatives, etc)

F50.2 Bulimia Nervosa
- Binge eating with minimal sense of control
- Purging or over exercising

F50.81 Binge Eating Disorder
- Binge eating with minimal sense of control
- No purging or over exercising to try to compensate

FEEDING DISORDERS

F50.82 Avoidant / Restrictive Food Intake Disorder
- Extreme food preferences leading to substantial psychosocial or nutritional problems

F98.3 Pica (children)
F50.8 Pica (adults)
- Eating non-food items for 1 month or more
- Inappropriate for age

F98.21 Rumination Disorder
- Persistent regurgitation of food (may be re-chewed or spit out)

ELIMINATION DISORDERS

F98.0 Enuresis - Loss of control of urine, age 5 or older

F98.1 Encopresis - Loss of control of feces, age 4 or older

NEUROCOGNITIVE DISORDERS

F05 Delirium
- Quick onset disturbance in attention, orientation, and cognition (memory, language & perception)
- Evidence of a medical cause (substance intoxication or withdrawal, toxin, medication reaction, or other physical illness)
- May also be more specific in coding to specific cause

R41.9 Major Neurocognitive Disorder
- Significant cognitive decline in one or more areas (learning and memory, language, executive functioning, complex attention, perceptual-motor, or social cognition)
- Interferes to the point of needing assistance
- Specify (and code) subtypes when possible: Alzheimer's, Vascular, Substance Induced, Traumatic Brain Injury, HIV, Parkinson's Disease, Lewy Bodies, Prion Disease, Huntington's Disease, and Frontotemporal Degneration

Specify:
Mild, Moderate or Severe
With Behavioral Disturbance
Without Behavioral Disturbance

Mild Neurocognitive Disorders
- Modest cognitive decline in one or more areas (learning and memory, language, executive functioning, complex attention, perceptual-motor, or social cognition)
- Does not interfere with functioning or independence
- Specify (and code) subtypes when possible: Alzheimer's, Vascular, Substance Induced, Traumatic Brain Injury, HIV, Parkinson's Disease, Lewy Bodies, Prion Disease, Huntington's Disease, and Frontotemporal Degneration

Specify:
With Behavioral Disturbance
Without Behavioral Disturbance

DISRUPTIVE IMPULSE-CONTROL DISORDERS

F91.3 Oppositional Defiant Disorder
- Angry, argumentative, vindictive or defiant behavior for 6 months
- Marked distress or impairment

F91.9 Conduct Disorder
- Persistently violates other's rights or societal rules (hurting people or animals, property destruction, lying, theft, illegal activity)
- May code more specifically for Childhood or Adolescent onset

F63.81 Intermittent Explosive Disorder
- Recurrent verbal or physical outbursts out of character for the person and disproportionate to the stress

F63.2 Kleptomania
- Recurrent impulsive stealing of un-needed items
- Build up of tension prior to the act and relief following it

F63.1 Pyromania
- Recurrent fire setting and attraction to fire
- Buildup of tension prior to the act and relief following it

SOMATIC DISORDERS

F45.1 Somatic Symptom Disorder
- Disproportionately excessive response (thoughts, feelings or behaviors) to a distressing physical symptom
- Usually persists at least 6 months

F45.21 Illness Anxiety Disorder
- Excessive worry over having a serious illness, despite minimal medical evidence
- High anxiety around health overall
- Excessive health-related activities (symptom checking, tests, doctor visits, etc.), or avoids medical care

F54 Psychological Factors Affecting Medical Condition
- Psychological factors adversely affect the course of a medical illness

F68.10 Factitious Disorder
- Intentional faking to achieve a sick role
- No clear economic or legal motivators

F44.x Functional Neurological Symptom Disorder (Conversion Disorder)
- Abnormal voluntary motor or sensory functioning
- Symptoms are incompatible with recognized neurologic or medical conditions
- Marked distress or impairment

> Document Subtype:
> F44.4: Weakness, paralysis, abnormal movement, swallowing, speech
> F44.5: Seizures
> F44.6: Anesthesia or sensory loss
> F44.7: Mixed

SLEEP-WAKE DISORDERS

F51.01 Insomnia Disorder
- Difficulty initiating or maintaining sleep, 3 nights a week for at least 3 months
- Marked distress or impairment

F51.11 Hypersomnolence Disorder
- Excessive sleepiness despite sleeping at least 7 hours per night
- One of the following: non-restorative sleep lasting 9 hours or more, recurrent lapsing into sleep through the day, or difficulty awakening
- Occurs 3 times a week for at least 3 months
- Marked distress or impairment
- Not better explained by: sleep apnea, narcolepsy, parasomnias etc.

Narcolepsy
- Irresistible sleep attacks, at least 3 times a week for 3 months
- At least one of the following:
  - Cataplexy: sudden loss of muscle tone after laughing
  - Hypocretin deficiency on spinal tap
  - Sleep study showing reduced REM sleep latency
- DSM-5 coded by specific subtypes

G47.2x Circadian Rhythm Sleep-Wake Disorders
G47.21 - Delayed Sleep Phase
G47.22 - Advanced Sleep Phase
G47.23 - Irregular Sleep-wake Type
G47.24 - Non 24-hour Sleep-wake Type
G47.26 - Shift work type
G47.20 - Unspecified type

BREATHING RELATED SLEEP DISORDERS

G47.33 Obstructive Sleep Apnea Hypopnea
- Diagnosed via sleep study

G47.31 Central Sleep Apnea
- Diagnosed via sleep study
- ICD 10 coded by specific subtypes

G47.34 Sleep-Related Hypoventilation
- Diagnosed via sleep study
- ICD 10 coded by specific subtypes

PARASOMNIAS

F51.5 Nightmare Disorder
- Repeated terrifying awakenings with vivid recall and alertness
- Marked distress or impairment

G47.52 Rapid Eye Movement Sleep Behavior Disorder
- Repeated sleep arousals with speaking or complex movements (walking, etc.)
- Awakens, alert, and not disoriented

G25.81 Restless Legs Syndrome
- Urges to move legs, unpleasant restless sensation in legs, worse at night
- Occur at least 3 times a week for 3 months
- Marked distress or impairment

Non-REM Sleep Arousal Disorders
- No or little dream material recalled

F51.3 Sleepwalking type: blank stare, relatively unresponsive, hard to awaken, no dream recall

F51.4 Sleep Terror type: abrupt arousals, panic scream, intense fear and autonomic arousal

GENDER DYSPHORIA

Gender Dysphoria
- Incongruence between one's assigned gender and their experience of their gender. A strong preference for characteristics of the opposite gender to which they were assigned.
- Clinically significant distress or impairment
- In Children - **F64.2**
- In Adolescence / Adults - **F64.0**

SEXUAL DISORDERS

F52.22 Female Sexual Interest / Arousal Disorder
- Absent or reduced sexual interest or arousal

F52.21 Erectile Disorder

F52.31 Female Orgasmic Disorder
- Delayed or absence of orgasm

F52.32 Delayed Ejaculation

F52.6 Genito-Pelvic Pain/Penetration Disorder

F52.0 Male Hypoactive Sexual Desire Disorder

F52.4 Premature (Early) Ejaculation

PARAPHILIC DISORDERS

F65.2 Exhibitionistic Disorder
- Fantasies or behavior to expose genitals to unsuspecting others
- Marked distress or impairment

F65.0 Fetishistic Disorder
- Intense sexual fantasies or behavior with non-living object or non-genital body part
- Marked distress or impairment

F65.4 Pedophilic Disorder
- Fantasies or behavior of sexual activity with a prepubescent child (usually 13 and under)
- The perpetrator is 16 years of age or older, and is 5 years older than victim
- Marked distress or impairment

F65.81 Frotteuristic Disorder
- Fantasies or behaviors of touching or rubbing again an unsuspecting adult
- Marked distress or impairment

F65.52 Sexual Sadism Disorder
- Fantasies or behaviors of inflicting suffering on others

F65.51 Sexual Masochism Disorder
- Fantasies or behaviors of experiencing sexual humiliation or suffering
- Marked distress or impairment

F65.1 Transvestic Disorder
- Fantasies or behaviors of cross-dressing
- Marked distress or impairment

F65.3 Voyeuristic Disorder
- Arousal from observing unsuspecting person in sexual context or disrobed
- Marked distress or impairment

F65.89 Other Specified Paraphilic Disorder
Other paraphilias such as telephone scatologia (obscene calls), necrophilia (dead body), zoophilia (animals), coprophilia (feces), klismaphilia (enemas), urophilia, etc.
- Marked distress or impairment

PERSONALITY DISORDERS

CLUSTER A: "ODD" GROUP

F60.0 Paranoid Personality Disorder
- Distrust since early adulthood
- 4 out of 7 symptoms: suspects deception, doubts loyalty of friends, reluctant to confide, reads hidden meanings, bears grudges, perceives personal attacks on character, unwarranted suspicions of partner

F60.1 Schizoid Personality Disorder
- Detached social relationships
- 4 out of 7 symptoms: doesn't desire close relationships, solitary activities, no interest in a sex partner, few close friends, little pleasure in activities, indifferent to praise or criticism, emotional coldness or flat affect

F21 Schizotypal Personality Disorder
- Eccentricities and few close relationships
- 5 out of 9 symptoms: odd behavior, magical thinking (ESP, superstitions), ideas of reference, illusions, odd thinking and speech, paranoia, inappropriate or constricted affect, few close friends, excessive social anxiety

CLUSTER B: "DRAMATIC" GROUP

F60.3 Borderline Personality Disorder
- Unstable relationships, unstable self-image, unstable affects and impulsivity
- 5 out of 9 symptoms: frantically avoids abandonment, idealizes then devalues relationships, identity disturbance, dangerous impulsivity, recurrent suicidal thoughts or self-mutilation, affective instability, chronic empty feeling, anger control problems, transient dissociation or paranoia

F60.4 Histrionic Personality Disorder
- Excessive emotions and attention seeking
- 5 out of 8 symptoms: center of attention, sexually seductive, shallow and unstable emotions, dresses to draw attention, emotional speech without substance, theatrical, suggestible and easily influenced, feels relationships are more intimate than they really are

F60.81 Narcissistic Personality Disorder
- Grandiosity, need for admiration and lack of empathy since early adulthood
- 5 out of 9 symptoms: grandiosity, fantasies of unlimited power and success, sees self as "special" and only associates with others of high status, needs admiration, sense of entitlement, interpersonally exploitative, lacks empathy, envious of others, arrogant

F60.2 Antisocial Personality Disorder
- Evidence of conduct disorder before age 15
- Disregards other's rights since age 15
- 3 out of 7 symptoms: repeated unlawful acts, deceitfulness, impulsivity, repeated physical fights, disregard for safety, consistent irresponsibility, lack of remorse

CLUSTER C: "WITHDRAWN" GROUP

F60.6 Avoidant Personality Disorder
- Inhibited, inadequate and hypersensitive
- 4 out of 7 symptoms: avoids occupations dealing with people, avoids people unless they'll be liked, restrained in close relationships, fears social rejection, social inhibition, feels socially inept, few new activities or risks

F60.7 Dependent Personality Disorder
- Excessive need to be taken care of
- Submissive and clingy behavior
- Fears of separation
- 5 out of 8 symptoms: difficulty making decisions, doesn't take responsibility, avoids conflict, poor initiation of projects, craves nurturance, helpless when alone, urgently seeks out relationships when one ends, fears being left to take care of themselves

F60.5 Obsessive-Compulsive Personality Disorder
- Orderly, perfectionistic and in control
- 4 out of 8 symptoms: overly preoccupied by details; interfering perfectionism, workaholic, overly strict values, pack rat, micromanages others, miserly, rigid and stubborn

SECTION I
OVERVIEW

CHAPTER 1

INTRODUCTION

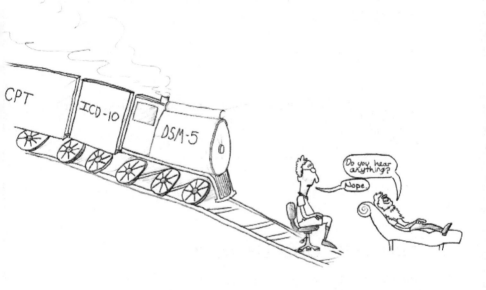

This book is for busy clinicians wishing to get a quick command and overview of the *Diagnostic and Statistical Manual of Mental Disorders, Fifth Edition, Text Revision (DSM-5-TR)*. The audience for this book includes therapists, psychiatrists, psychologists, counselors, physicians, residents in training, medical students, others in the mental health field, and interested laypersons.

We make liberal use of cartoons and hyperbole to capture broad ideas. We ask the reader's indulgence; we recognize that these conventions do not capture the nuance and subtle features that so often accompany people into the consulting room. The authors hope that by presenting engaging cartoons that attempt to reduce complex ideas into easily remembered images, the process of transition from earlier versions of the DSM to the present one, DSM-5-TR, will be made easier.

Throughout this book, certain conventions are used to assist the reader in remembering principles and ideas.

 This signifies a newly created diagnosis or category.

 This signifies that diagnoses or categories have been condensed/compressed.

This signifies an expansion of a category.

 This signifies that something has been moved (often unchanged).

~~~~~~~~~~~~~~~~~

I'm interested in themes that endure from generation to generation.

DAVID GUTERSON

GENERATIONS OF DSM

The DSM-5-TR was released nine years after the DSM-5, which itself arrived 20 years after its predecessor, the DSM-IV. That is a generation in the human family. The DSM-IV had embedded itself in the fabric of how mental illness was conceptualized and reshaped the boundary between mental health and mental illness.

The DSM-5-TR remains a symptom-driven system of classification. At the *National Institute of Mental Health*, there continue to be those who seek to move away from the DSM's symptom-based approach in favor of a greater focus on biology, genetics, and neuroscience (i.e., a causal approach).[1]

According to Thomas Insel,

We are committed to new and better treatments, but we feel this will only happen by developing a more precise diagnostic system.[2]

This book provides a conceptual framework whereby mental illness is understood to exist along a continuum of severity and presenting symptoms. We propose eight key groupings of mental illness that easily lend themselves to this *Spectrum* approach. Within each grouping, a spectrum of severity and functioning is presented. Each *Spectrum* is depicted with a mnemonic device and a cartoon. The cartoon captures a fundamental idea, *enantiodroma*, that was introduced to modern psychology by the Swiss psychiatrist Carl Gustav Jung. *Enantiodromia* is "the emergence of the unconscious opposite over time."[3] The extreme end of a *Spectrum* can be understood to evoke its opposite in the unconscious. These opposite ends of any *Spectrum* bookend a middle region where extremes become tempered, and balance is achieved.[4]

Chapter 2 begins with a historical overview of DSM-5-TR. Chapters 3 and 4 review what is new in DSM-5-TR, while also covering the major changes from DSM-IV that were introduced to DSM-5 in 2013. These chapters emphasize the idea that mental disorders exist along a *Spectrum*. For example, *Bipolar Disorder* is no longer conceived of just as a neatly defined disorder with a set of discrete signs and symptoms. In earlier versions of the DSM, patients either met criteria or they failed to meet criteria for a diagnosis. This approach led some clinicians to embellish findings to ensure a patient met diagnostic criteria. Alternatively, some clinicians tended to ignore certain criteria in an effort to assign a patient more benign-appearing diagnoses than might have been warranted by strict adherence to a set of enumerated criteria.

Chapter 5 presents the central idea of this book, namely the *8 Primary Spectrums of Mental Illness*. These *8 Spectrums* are covered in more detail in Chapters 6 through 13 (one chapter for each of the *Spectrums*). They provide a simplified, useful, and practical framework for clinicians to understand the DSM-5-TR's spectrum approach to diagnosis. For example, when considering *Bipolarity*, a person situated at the extreme end of the spectrum will demonstrate a full complement of symptoms associated with *Bipolar Affective Disorder* in the manic phase (see Chapter 7). At the other extreme of *Bipolarity*, a depressed person would be noted to be thoroughly lacking in creativity, risk-taking, and verve.

A cartoon caricature depicting each of the *8 Spectrums of Mental Illnesses* is intended to anchor in the reader's memory the most prominent features associated with various diagnostic categories. Healthy, well-balanced psychological functioning tends to be found in the middle of each spectrum.

Chapter 14 addresses many, but not all, of the remaining diagnoses that appear in DSM-5-TR. These diagnoses are neither less important nor less disruptive to the sufferer than the diagnoses presented within the *8 Spectrums of Mental Illness*. However, apart from Trauma, the disorders covered in Chapter 14 may simply occur less frequently, or clinicians may be less likely to encounter these disorders in daily practice. Furthermore, many of these disorders do not lend themselves easily to the spectrum approach put forth in the DSM-5-TR. The convention of using a scale of severity has not been extended as much to the conditions covered in Chapter 14. The Chapter 14 disorders *include Trauma- and Stressor-Related Disorders, Dissociative Disorders, Somatic Symptom and Related Disorders, Feeding and Eating Disorders, Elimination Disorders, Sleep-Wake Disorders, Sexual Dysfunctions, Gender Dysphoria, Neurocognitive Disorders,* and *Paraphilic Disorders.*

While DSM-5-TR does not formally recognize trauma as a spectrum phenomenon, the authors have speculated how trauma might be within a *spectrum* approach.

Chapter 15, *The Harmony of the Lotus Flower*, emerges from the concept of the *8 Spectrums of Mental Illness*. By overlaying each of the *8 Primary Spectrums of Mental Illness* over one another, an image of a lotus flower is produced. At the center exists an idealized realm, in which each of the spectrums achieves a balance. In this domain, one's inner and outer life display greater harmony between opposing forces. This chapter is unabashedly Jungian in its perspective. It proposes a conjunction of opposites within the psyche, a *conjunctio oppositurum* according to Jungian psychology. It permits an individual to fluidly move between the best aspects of each of the extremes, with confidence knowing that it is balanced and tempered by its opposite. Chaos and symptoms emerge on the periphery of the lotus flower. In contrast, movement toward the center results in balance, adaptability, and fuller expressions of the *Archetypal Self.*

Modern physics has revealed that at the subatomic level, a precise determination of a particle's position and velocity cannot be made. This principle of *uncertainty* fits nicely with the elusive exercise of establishing a diagnosis. It reminds all clinicians that we can never locate a person with complete precision. Perhaps to fix a person diagnostically makes a person's individual narrative more imprecise, whereas a singular focus on the details of a person's unique story fails to locate them within a commonly recognized diagnostic schema. Once again, what is required is a balance between such extremes.

Chapter 16 offers another Jungian perspective on DSM-5-TR. We indulge in a bit of *active imagination* of our own in which Jung is confronted with DSM-5-TR. It should be kept in mind that Jung began his career as a researcher using the word association test. These pioneering efforts to study the responses evoked by certain words, aided his understanding of the unconscious.

Lastly, the appendix introduces ICD-10 codes that apply to psychiatry, psychology, and other mental health disciplines. ICD-10 uses three to seven digits instead of the three to five digits used with the prior ICD-9, as the coding is more specific in ICD-10.

CHAPTER 2

THE HISTORY OF THE DSM

Early efforts to systematically classify mental illness were present in antiquity. To varying degrees these systems tended to emphasize presenting symptoms, presumed causes, and distinguishing features between disorders. Because different systems of diagnosis and nomenclature emphasized different things, translation between different systems proved difficult. *DSM-5-TR Insanely Simplified: Unlocking the Spectrums within DSM-5 & ICD-10* preserves the effort to make the transition between DSM-IV and DSM-5 easier while incorporating the changes introduced in the DSM-5-TR. A fundamental shift occurred from DSM-IV to DSM-5 through the introduction of the concept of diagnoses along a spectrum. A brief history of different systems of classification of mental disorders is a helpful starting place.

ANTIQUITY

Hippocrates recognized distinct categories of mental illness that included melancholia, mania, and paranoia. An ancient theory of causation was that "imbalances of humors" produced mental disturbances.

PERSIA AND THE MUSLIM EMPIRE

Arabic and Persian scholars translated the works of the Greeks and Romans. These scholars expanded the diagnostic categories to include delusional disorders, anger, aggression, and other disorders. The Holy Qur'an advises against entrusting to the *insane* material belongings given by Allah, but it goes on to instruct that such persons be fed and clothed with the property that belongs to them.[5] The first psychiatric hospital was established in Baghdad in 705 AD. The cause of mental illness was often thought to be *Jinn*, spiritual creatures capable of possessing a person.

EARLY CHRISTENDOM

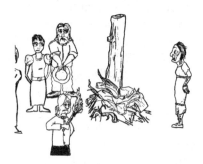

While early European Christendom distinguished between *idiocy* and *lunacy*, causation was commonly ascribed to evil forces. By the close of the 17th century, mental illness was being recognized as an organic disorder. Nevertheless, madhouses continued to treat their inmates like wild beasts in need of taming. Bedlam, the most notorious of the madhouses, went so far as to charge spectators for the privilege of watching the inmates.

19TH CENTURY AND BEYOND

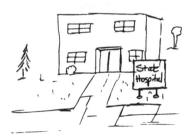

Dorothea Dix campaigned for better treatment of the mentally ill. She petitioned the government of the United States to build large institutions to house people with mental disorders. Eventually, 32

state psychiatric hospitals were established around the country. The 19th century also witnessed the introduction of familiar terms like obsession neurosis, agoraphobia, somatization disorder, kleptomania, pyromania, and psychopathic inferiority.

STATISTICAL MANUAL FOR THE USE OF INSTITUTIONS FOR THE INSANE (1844-1917)

Beginning in 1844, the forerunner of the *American Psychiatric Association* compiled statistical information about patients living in mental institutions around the nation. In 1917, a committee on statistics produced a report that included 22 separate diagnoses.

DSM-I RELEASED IN 1952 (ORIGINAL PRICE $3.90)

The first DSM was produced in 1952 and was based largely on the nomenclature used by psychiatrists in World War II. It attempted to ensure that DSM diagnoses conformed to the *International Classification of Diseases-6th Edition* (ICD-6). The first DSM-1 was 130 pages in length and included 106 mental disorders. It introduced the idea of "reaction," in part, due to the influence of Adolph Meyer, a University of Zurich-trained American psychiatrist who advanced the notion of a biopsychosocial model of understanding psychopathology. The DSM-I distinguished personality disturbance from neurosis.

DSM-II RELEASED IN 1968

The DSM-II expanded the number of diagnoses to 182. The DSM-II tried to strive toward an "atheoretical" approach. However, vestiges of classical psychoanalysis and psychodynamic theory were evident in the broad distinction made between neurosis and psychosis. The DSM-II was designed to conform to ICD-8.

DSM-II harked back to antiquity, when homosexuality had been referred to as *Scythians Disease*. Herodotus twice mentioned *enareë*, male diviners possessed by Aphrodite who displayed androgenous, nonbinary traits.[6] In DSM-II homosexuality was considered a Mental Disorder. This changed in 1974.

DSM-III RELEASED IN 1980 (ORIGINAL PRICE $25.00)

The DSM-III introduced the multiaxial system of diagnoses and conformed to ICD-9.

The Multiaxial System included:
Axis I: Clinical Disorders of Mental Illness
Axis II: Personality Disorders and Mental Retardation
Axis III: General Medical Conditions
Axis IV: Psychosocial and Environmental Problems
          (homelessness, legal issues, etc.)
Axis V: Global Assessment of Functioning:
          A single number from O to 100

There was a clear shift away from a psychodynamic approach and a biopsychosocial model rose to prominence. The DSM-III grew to 494 pages and recognized 265 diagnoses. One shortcoming of the DSM-III was its all-or-nothing approach to diagnosis. A specific number of symptoms had to be met in order to meet criteria to establish a diagnosis.

DSM-III-R RELEASED IN 1987

This revision made modest changes in the organization of DSM-III and made changes in criteria. Additionally, the number of diagnoses rose to 292, and the book expanded to 567 pages.

DSM-IV RELEASED IN 1994 (ORIGINAL PRICE $65.00)

The DSM-IV changed very little; nevertheless, it expanded to 886 pages and added five more disorders to reach a total of 297 disorders. It conformed to ICD-9. Considerable controversy was provoked by the publication of DSM-III earlier, and this led to an exhaustive amount of literature review, extensive review of data compiled using DSM-III, and 13 work groups were called upon to manage specific sections of DSM-IV.

DSM-IV-TR RELEASED IN 2000 (ORIGINAL PRICE $84.00)

DSM-IV-TR "Text Revision" corrected significant errors and improved the supportive educational material. It also made some additional refinements to assure conformity with the ICD-9 system.

DSM-5 RELEASED IN 2013 (ORIGINAL PRICE $199.00)

The work to revise DSM-IV began in 1999. Once again, 13 working groups were established. An enormous amount of money, $3 million, was spent on what proved to be mostly useless field testing. The thrust of DSM-5 was designed to usher in a system of classification whereby mental disorders were understood to exist along a spectrum. DSM-5 strove to be more evidence-based. There was an attempt to eliminate the category of *Not Otherwise Specified (NOS)*. DSM-5 appeared just prior to the release dates of ICD-10. The transition from ICD-9 to ICD-10 was delayed until 2015; therefore, both codes appeared in DSM-5. The DSM-5 was 992 pages in length.

DSM-5-TR RELEASED IN 2022 (PRICE IN HARDCOVER: $220.00)

DSM-5-TR was released in March of 2022 and contains a number of revisions. Pertinent social issues were reevaluated, including extensive literature reviews and language updates on gender and racial issues. Several diagnostic criteria were modified and a new diagnosis, *Prolonged Grief Disorder*, was added.

The DSM has been, and likely will continue to be, an amalgam of theoretical concepts, social mores, and evidence-based contributions intended to serve multiple purposes. It introduced a degree of diagnostic uniformity for researchers and clinicians. It sometimes codified social constructs like *Masochistic Personality Disorder* that was added in DSM-III and subsequently removed in DSM-IV. One lasting impact of the DSM-III and its successors is that it became the standard diagnostic categorization upon which insurance reimbursement was based.

CHAPTER 3

WHAT IS NEW IN DSM-5-TR?

The changes introduced in DSM-5-TR are modest in scope and not nearly as transformative as when DSM-5 replaced DSM-IV. DSM-5-TR preserves the spectrum approach of its predecessor, while introducing important updates and modifications. Pertinent social issues have been reevaluated, including extensive literature reviews and language updates on gender and racial issues. Diagnostic criteria have been modified for more than 70 mental health disorders. DSM-5-TR introduces symptom codes for suicidal behavior and non-suicidal self-injury. *Unspecified Mood Disorder,* which was removed in DSM-5, was restored in DSM-5-TR, and a new diagnosis of *Prolonged Grief Disorder* was added. The descriptive text was reviewed and updated.

PROLONGED GRIEF DISORDER

In the past, clinicians have struggled with how to characterize marked depressive symptoms in the context of profound bereavement. Bereavement shares many features with depressive disorders. It was often thought that this was a "normal depression" and shouldn't be diagnosed. Often the only category that seemed to fit was *Other Specified Trauma and Stressor-Related Disorder* (F43.8). This often proved inadequate. DSM-5-TR remedied this by adding the diagnosis *Prolonged Grief Disorder*. It pertains to intense yearning or preoccupation of the deceased loved one beyond one year from their death. Three or more emotional symptoms are required as well. One in 10 adults are at risk for developing *Prolonged Grief Disorder* after the death of a loved one. Below is a summary of the new criteria.

F43.8 PROLONGED GRIEF DISORDER

- Death of a loved one, 1 year ago or more (6 months for children)
- Near-constant intense yearning or preoccupation with memories of deceased
- Significant distress
- 3 or more symptoms most days of: loneliness, meaninglessness, emotional numbness, identity disruption, denial of the loved one's death, avoiding reminders, intense emotional pain, or being unable to resume with activities and friends

UNSPECIFIED MOOD DISORDER

Unspecified Mood Disorder had been removed from the DSM-IV. This proved to be problematic for some providers, particularly when mood symptoms did not fall clearly within depression or bipolar criteria. ***Unspecified Mood Disorder*** allows the diagnosis to maintain this level of uncertainty, yet still document the mood symptoms.

DIAGNOSTIC CRITERIA

Diagnostic criteria have been revised for numerous diagnoses. These include *Major Depressive Disorder, Persistent Depressive Disorder, Manic Episodes, Bipolar I* and *Bipolar II disorders, Cyclothymic Disorder, PTSD* (in children), *Autism Spectrum Disorder, Avoidant-Restrictive Food In- take Disorder,* and *Delirium.*

Please see the DSM-5-TR summary pages in the beginning of this book for full details.

REVISED CODING

New and revised coding is now in place in DSM-5-TR for:
- *Substance Use Disorders*
- *Neurocognitive Disorders*
- *Suicidal Behavior*
- *Non-suicidal Self-Injury*

REVISED NOMENCLATURE

The diagnoses and phrases revised in the DSM-5-TR include:
- *Experienced gender* replaces *Desired gender*
- *Gender-affirming medical procedure* replaces *Cross-sex medical procedure*
- *Individual assigned male/female at birth* replaces *Natal male/female*
- *Intellectual Developmental Disorder* replaces *Intellectual Disability*
- *Functional Neurological Symptom Disorder* replaces *Conversion Disorder*
- *Antipsychotic medication* replaces *Neuroleptic*

CHAPTER 4

WHAT WAS NEW IN DSM-5?

One of the major shifts from DSM-IV to DSM-5 was the removal of the *Multi-axial System of Diagnosis* (Axis I, II, III, IV, V). In its place came a conceptual model of mental illness along a spectrum of severity that gave more emphasis to a developmental approach.

Woven into the very fabric of DSM-5 was this concept of a s*pectrum* of functioning and severity, from very minimal or "normal" levels to more extreme "pathologic" symptoms.

DSM-5 made a less clear distinction between "normal" and "mentally ill." It utilized two new terms, *Subtypes* and *Specifiers,* to further refine diagnostic impressions.

DSM-5 introduced several other changes as well. The following are some of the highlights:

DEPRESSION

> *"In depression this faith in deliverance, in ultimate restoration, is absent. The pain is unrelenting, and what makes the condition intolerable is the foreknowledge that no remedy will come — not in a day, an hour, a month, or a minute.; (…)"*
>
> William Styron[7]

Depression has been described as the *gout of the soul*. Like gout, it recurs, it causes intense discomfort, and in between flare-ups, little evidence that it ever visited may be present. However, DSM-III introduced the diagnosis of *Dysthymic Disorder* or

Dysthymia. This term, *Dysthymia,* coined by Dr. Robert Spitzer, who chaired the task force that developed DSM-III, replaced the psychoanalytically oriented term *neurotic depression.* It established a diagnosis for chronic, unrelenting, milder forms of depression. Years later, Dr. Spitzer expressed reservations about how DSM-III had medicalized the normal human experience.

The distinguishing feature of *Dysthymic Disorder* was a depressive disorder lasting at least two years that failed to meet the full criteria for *Major Depression. Persistent Depressive Disorder* replaced the previous DSM-IV diagnosis of *Dysthymic Disorder.* With DSM-5, both *Dysthymic Disorder* and *Recurrent (Chronic) Major Depression* were consolidated under a single, newly created diagnosis. The result is that the persistent quality of the depression replaces severity as a defining feature.

The *Mixed Features Specifiers* allow clinicians to document the presence of significant *bipolarity.* Similarly, the *Anxiety Specifiers* allow significant anxiety components to be documented. In earlier versions of the DSM, the presence of bereavement excluded the diagnosis of depression; this is no longer the case. Patients who are actively grieving may be diagnosed with depression. Finally, DSM-5 introduced a new disorder to this category, *Premenstrual Dysphoric Disorder.*

BIPOLAR DISORDER

Greater emphasis was placed upon *increased energy* and *increased activity level* with less emphasis being given to whether or not there appear features like expansiveness, euphoria, and irritability. The Bipolar diagnosis can include *Mixed Features Specifiers* that allow clinicians to document significant *Depressive* and *Anxiety* features.

ANXIETY DISORDERS

DSM-5 removed *Obsessive Compulsive Disorder (OCD)* and *Post Traumatic Stress Disorder (PTSD)* from the section of *Anxiety Disorders.* They were then placed among two newly created categories, *OCD and Related Disorders* and *Trauma Stress Disorders*, respectively.

DSM-5 distinguished *Panic Disorder* and *Agoraphobia* as two distinct disorders. Recognizing that panic attacks appear in the presence of various other disorders, clinicians may use a *Panic Attack Specifier*. This also makes clear that a panic attack is not a mental disorder, per se.

PSYCHOSIS

The five subtypes of *Schizophrenia* (*catatonic, disorganized, paranoid, residual*, and *undifferentiated*) no longer characterized this disorder. Instead, *Catatonia* became a *Specifier* and could be employed with *Schizophrenia, Bipolar Disorder*, and *Depression*. At least one positive symptom (hallucinations, delusions, or disorganized speech) was now required to meet the criteria for *Schizophrenia*. *Schizoaffective Disorder* required that either depression or bipolar features be present for most of the disorder's duration.

OBSESSIVE COMPULSIVE AND RELATED DISORDERS

DSM-5 added a new group of disorders known as the *OCD and Related Disorders* that, in addition to OCD, included *Body Dysmorphic Disorder* and *Trichotillomania*. Newly created diagnoses in this section were *Excoriation Disorder* (skin picking) and *Hoarding Disorder*.

SUBSTANCE ABUSE DISORDERS

The distinction between *Substance Abuse* and *Substance Dependence* was eliminated in keeping with the "*Spectrum*" approach. The main diagnostic heading became *Substance Abuse Disorders*.

Severity was associated with the number of diagnostic criteria met, and the criteria were grouped as seen below.

Criteria 1-4	Related to cravings and overuse
Criteria 5-7	Impaired social functioning
Criteria 8-9	Failure to consider risks of use
Criterion 10	Tolerance
Criterion 11	Withdrawal

DSM-5 recognized cravings as a hallmark feature of *Substance Use Disorders*, and the first group of Criteria 1-4 reflects this. Impaired social functioning is established with Criteria 5-7. The failure to consider the risks of use is reflected in Criteria 8-9. Criterion 10 addresses tolerance—the phenomenon whereby an increasing dose of a substance is required to produce a desired effect. Criterion 11 addresses withdrawal—the physiologic phenomenon whereby symptoms arise upon abrupt cessation of a substance after prolonged use. Note that neither tolerance nor withdrawal is required to establish the diagnosis. The criterion of "recurrent substance-related legal problems" was removed.

Substances of abuse include *Alcohol, Caffeine, Cannabis, Hallucinogens, Opioids, Sedative-Hypnotics/Anxiolytics, Stimulants, Tobacco,* and *Other*. Though many designer drugs can be subsumed under some of these headings, the *Other* category may become increasingly important as new/emerging psychoactive substances appear.

The severity may be described as *mild, moderate,* or *severe,* depending upon the number of criteria that are met. Clinicians can specify whether *intoxication* or *withdrawal* is involved.

Tobacco Use Disorder has also been added.

Gambling Disorder was recognized in DSM-5 as sharing sufficient features in common with *Substance Use Disorders* to warrant inclusion in this category as well.

NEURODEVELOPMENTAL DISORDERS

The *Neurodevelopmental Disorders* first appear in childhood and are capable of producing lasting impairment of academic, social, occupational, and interpersonal functioning. The disorders include: *Autism Spectrum Disorder (ASD), Attention Deficit Hyperactivity Disorder (ADHD), Communication Disorder, Specific Learning Disorder,* and *Motor Disorders.*

 DSM-5 combined *Autism, Asperger's Disorder, Childhood Disintegrative Disorder,* and *Pervasive Developmental Disorder NOS* into one diagnosis called *Autism Spectrum Disorder (ASD). Asperger's Disorder,* previously viewed as less stigmatizing, was now officially an *ASD.*

ASD is characterized by 1) deficits in social communication and social interaction and 2) restricted repetitive behaviors. Where only social communication and interaction are impaired, the diagnosis should be *Social Communication Disorder.*

Specific Learning Disorder replaced *Reading Disorder, Mathematics Disorder,* and *Disorder of Written Expression,* while clinicians could still specify if any of those features were present.

The diagnosis of *Mental Retardation* was replaced by *Intellectual Developmental Disorder,* which was assessed more by adaptive functioning and less by absolute IQ score.

PERSONALITY DISORDERS

While DSM-5 abolished Axis II, it did not remove the personality disorders. Instead, these diagnoses were simply listed like any other disorder. The criteria for personality disorders were virtually unchanged in DSM-5. All 10 personality disorders from DSM-IV were carried over into DSM-5.

TRAUMA-RELATED DISORDERS

NEW — DSM-5 established a new section for *Trauma and Stressor Related Disorders*. This included: *PTSD, Acute Stress Disorder, Adjustment Disorders,* and *Reactive Attachment Disorder*. PTSD introduced a new cluster of symptoms pertaining to negative changes in an individual's mood and cognition, namely "Negative alterations in cognitions and mood associated with the traumatic event."[8] This addressed the features of lacunae (holes) in memory about traumatic events along with exaggeration, diminishing, distortion, and impaired emotional life that appear so commonly with trauma. Allowances were also made for indirect exposure to a traumatic event.

If dissociative symptoms are present, the clinician should specify with *Dissociative Symptoms*. Special mention is made for *Post-Traumatic Stress Disorder* for children 6 years and younger. *Adjustment disorder*, by definition results from stress and therefore was moved to the category of *Trauma- and Stressor-Related Disorders*.

NEUROCOGNITIVE DISORDERS

NEW — DSM-5 introduced a substantial shift in the diagnostic schema regarding *Dementia*. The term *Dementia* was replaced with *Neurocognitive Disorder (NCD)*. Here too, a spectrum of functioning is recognized by distinguishing *Mild NCDs* from *Major NCDs*. The *Neurocognitive Disorders* include a long list of subtypes based on the specific cause of the neurocognitive disorder. Subtypes include *Alzheimer's, Vascular, Substance Induced, Traumatic Brain Injury, HIV Infection, Parkinson's Disease, Lewy Bodies, Prion Disease,* and *Huntington's Disease*.

DISSOCIATIVE DISORDERS

Dissociative Disorders were listed as a separate diagnostic category that includes *Dissociative Identity Disorder* and *Dissociative Amnesia, Depersonalization/Derealization Disorder*. This last category replaced *Depersonalization Disorder* and joined it with the condition of derealization.

 Dissociative Fugue was no longer a distinct diagnosis but became available as a specifier.

SOMATIC SYMPTOM DISORDER

 Somatic Symptom Disorder was a new diagnostic construct in DSM-5. *Somatization Disorder, Hypochondriasis, Pain Disorder,* and *Undifferentiated Somatoform Disorder* were all removed and replaced by the new *Somatic Symptom Disorder* diagnosis. This disorder essentially considered the degree to which a patient with any physical symptoms was experiencing excessively distressing feelings, thoughts, or behaviors beyond what the physical symptoms would typically cause. This new diagnosis eliminated the requirement of "unexplained medical symptoms," which so often angered patients who felt they were being accused of "just making it up!" Furthermore, the diagnosis of somatoform disorder was more common with difficult-to-recognize conditions in which diagnosis could often be delayed.

FEEDING AND EATING DISORDERS

 This was new nomenclature in DSM-5. The diagnoses of *Pica* and *Rumination Disorder* were no longer restricted to childhood; the diagnosis could be assigned at any age. A new disorder,

Avoidant / Restrictive Food Intake Disorder, was primarily confined to children who had extreme food preferences leading to substantial psychological or nutritional problems. In women, *Anorexia Nervosa* no longer required amenorrhea. The frequency of purging behavior required to diagnose *Bulimia Nervosa* was reduced from twice per week to once per week. When overeating with a loss of control and significant distress occurred at least weekly for three months, a new disorder, *Binge-Eating Disorder* was introduced. Since the publication of DSM-5, some have argued that *Orthorexia Nervosa*, the pathologic obsession with eating food considered healthy, should be recognized as a separate disorder.[9]

SLEEP-WAKE DISORDER

Sleep disorders often arise in conjunction with other medical or neurological conditions. DSM-5 recommended "lumping them together" (as with insomnia) or "splitting them apart" (as with narcolepsy). *Primary Insomnia* was renamed *Insomnia Disorder*. Under the category of *Breathing-Related Sleep Disorders*, DSM-5 listed *Obstructive Sleep Apnea, Central Sleep Apnea,* and a new diagnosis of *Sleep-Related Hypoventilation*.

Other new sleep disorders included *Rapid Eye Movement Sleep Behavior Disorder* and *Restless Leg Syndrome*.

GENDER DYSPHORIA

Substantial changes have occurred in the attitudes toward persons who are Lesbian, Gay, Bisexual, Transgendered, Queer/Questioning, Intersex, Asexual, and more (LGBTQIA+) over the past 30 years since the release of DSM-IV. In fact, largely due to the efforts of Dr. Robert Spitzer, homosexuality was removed from DSM-III and was no longer considered to be a mental illness. *Gender Dysphoria* was no longer deemed an "identity disorder." Instead, dysphoria and difficulties in adapting were understood to be the result of gender incongruence. *Gender Dysphoria* was no longer grouped together with sexual dysfunctions and paraphilias. It was segregated into its own category. Controversy persisted, however, as one Brazilian author discouraged the use of DSM-5, citing the composition of the Working Group on Gender Dysphoria including members of five nationalities (US, Canada, Netherlands, UK, and Sweden) and no trans individuals.[10]

SEXUAL DYSFUNCTIONS

DSM-5 reorganized the section of *Sexual Dysfunctions* as well. *Genito-Pelvic Pain/Penetration Disorder* replaced *Vaginismus* and *Dyspareunia*. Furthermore, the diagnosis of *Sexual Aversion Disorder* was removed due to a lack of research evidence.

CHAPTER 5

8 PRIMARY PSYCHIATRIC SPECTRUMS OF MENTAL ILLNESS

A major shift occurred with the introduction of DSM-5 and subsequently DSM-5-TR that has broad implications for the way psychiatric illness is conceptualized. DSM-5 introduced the notion that illnesses exist along a spectrum or continuum rather than as discrete, either/or phenomena.

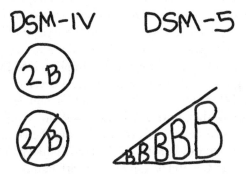

From the outset, the DSM-5 planning groups established the idea that throughout the new manual, the emphasis on illness as a spectrum would be apparent. Also, the boundaries between certain disorders are less sharply defined in DSM-5 and DSM-5-TR. For example, *Depression* can have *Bipolar* or *Anxiety* "specifiers," thereby acknowledging the overlap of the illness. Likewise, an *Anxiety Disorder* can be assigned *Bipolar* or *Depression* specifiers. *Autism Spectrum Disorder* incorporates this idea into its very name, thereby drawing attention away from the idea that separate, discrete disorders exist. Likewise, under the heading of *Substance Use Disorders*, both DSM-5 and DSM-5-TR use the number of criteria met to establish the level of severity rather than to simply determine the presence or absence of the disorder. Chapters 3 and 4 highlighted various examples where the concept of *illness along a spectrum* makes an appearance in DSM-5 and DSM-5-TR. This chapter takes this concept one step further by simplifying and encapsulating DSM-5-TR into the *8 Primary Spectrums of Psychiatry*.

CONSTRUCTING PRIMARY SPECTRUMS OF MENTAL ILLNESS

> *Everything should be made as simple as possible, but not simpler.*
> ALBERT EINSTEIN

We developed the *8 Primary Spectrums of Mental Illness* as a tool to improve understanding. The *Spectrums* are not strictly based upon a collection or grouping of symptoms in the style of DSM-IV. We recognize that a great deal of work was done to develop DSM-5 and DSM5-TR. Any attempt to simplify DSM5-TR risks undermining the considerable work done to develop it. However, the DSM-5-TR speaks for itself; this guide is intended to enhance the usefulness of the DSM-5-TR's rich content.

There is a real danger of oversimplifying the complexities of mental illness into tidy constructs. Diagnosis, like psychotherapy, is a *difficult art* and should be approached with humility and respect for the complexities of the human condition.[11] The following advice is offered:

> *The map is not the territory.*
> ALFRED KORZYBSKI

The clinician or layperson reading this book is advised to view these concepts broadly and cautiously. Beware to not impose them on patients. In making diagnoses, the clinician should avoid becoming like *Procrustes*, a rogue blacksmith who was intent on making travelers fit his iron bed by either stretching them or cutting off their legs. People are NOT their diagnoses.

Despite these pitfalls, the core constructs offered here may give clinicians an easy, big-picture approach to diagnosis along a spectrum as well as a means of monitoring the therapeutic process.

THE 8 PRIMARY SPECTRUMS OF MENTAL ILLNESS

The Depression Spectrum: Shallowness vs. Despair
The Mania Spectrum: Boring vs. Bipolar
The Anxiety Spectrum: Carelessness vs. Anxiousness
The Psychosis Spectrum: Visionless vs. Psychotic
The Focusing Spectrum: ADHD vs. OCD
The Substance Abuse Spectrum: Ascetic vs. Addicted
The Autism Spectrum: Codependent vs. Autistic
The Personality Spectrum: Neurotic vs. Obnoxious

Within each of these categories there exists a spectrum. At the extreme ends of each spectrum, problems emerge. The extreme ranges, where symptoms of mental illness appear, tend to interfere with life. The middle ranges of these spectrums are preferred. The authors' views are strongly influenced by the work of Dr. C. G. Jung and his idea of *coniunctio oppositorum*, meaning the psychological conjunction of opposites.

DSM-5-TR diagnosis concerns itself with the extreme ends of these spectrums. The middle of each spectrum is a zone of "healthy functioning." The power of this spectrum approach is that clinicians no longer are required to fit patients into either a category of "healthy" or "disordered." Instead, gradations along a spectrum encourage a more varied, nuanced understanding of the individual. The boundaries between normal and ill may become less clear, but clinicians are granted more latitude by being able to "specify" features that cross over from other diagnostic categories. When symptoms begin interfering with normal functioning, a sort of line is crossed that leads to diagnosis of an illness and treatment.

The question facing clinicians is no longer "Does a person have bipolar disorder or not?" but rather "How much bipolarity does a person have?" Everyone has some degree of bipolarity, for example, when overtaken by a surge of creativity, artistry, spontaneity, energy, sociability, talkativeness, or excitement. It is only when these features are "out of control," persistent, or produce negative consequences that a person enters the realm of what DSM-5-TR considers a "disorder."

Consider some ideas that derive from the concept of spectrums of illness.[12] How much *Depressive-ness* or *Introspective-ness* does a person have? How much *Anxious-ness, OCD-ness, ADD-ness, Psychotic-ness, Addicted-ness*, etc.

At first glance, it may seem that the ideal situation exists when a person shows as few characteristics as possible. However, the person displaying too few characteristics may have problems just like the person displaying excess. The *8 Primary Spectrums of Mental Illness* use a consistent convention whereby the left end of the spectrum represents a condition in which too few features are evident *(this is a problem)* and the right end of the spectrum represents a condition in which too many features or symptoms are present *(also a problem)*.

This concept often empowers patients suffering symptoms of mental illness. One implication of a spectrum approach is that features manifesting in extreme forms constitute symptoms, whereas in their attenuated form, the same features may be adaptive and desirable. "Normal" and "Abnormal" can be understood as states, not traits. This, in turn, may be less stigmatizing. The return to *normal* may appear more attainable.

Everyone falls somewhere along the eight spectrums. This conceptual model tends to destigmatize mental illness and strip it of shame. Just as the patient is located along a spectrum, so are other people in the patient's life. Everyone exists on a spectrum of severity or paucity of features. By highlighting what we have in common with those who suffer mental illness, the spectrums can reduce stigma and scapegoating.

Before proceeding to the more detailed presentation of the *8 Spectrums of Mental Illness,* spend a few minutes reflecting on the following eight illustrations. This will provide a visual introduction to the overarching concepts.

Shallowness vs. Despair
"How much SORROW do you hold?"

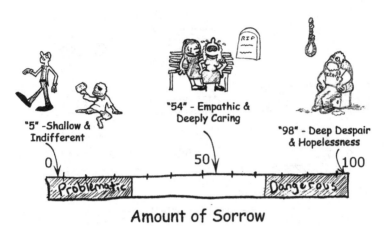

Amount of Sorrow

Boring vs. Bipolar
"How much CREATIVITY do you have?"

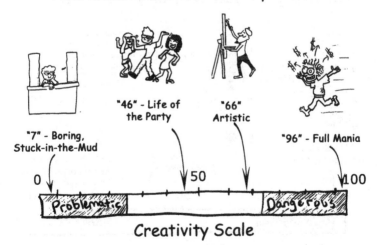

Creativity Scale

Carelessness vs. Anxiousness
"How much VIGILANCE do you have?"

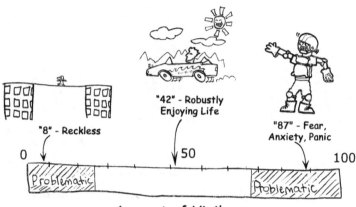

Amount of Vigilance

Visionless vs. Psychotic:
"How strong are your DREAMS and VISIONS?"

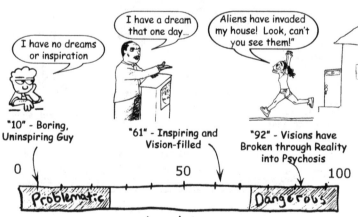

Intensity of Dreams and Visions

Attention Deficit Disorder (ADHD) vs. Obsessive Compulsive Disorder (OCD)
"How much FOCUS do you have?"

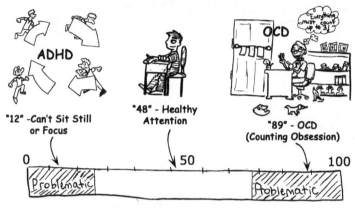

Amount of Focusing Ability

Ascetic Monk vs. Multiple Addictions:
"How Much PLEASURE Do You Seek?"

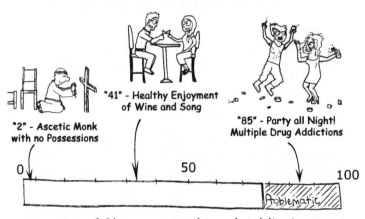

Amount of Pleasure Seeking / Addictiveness

Autism vs. Codependency:
How CONNECTED to Others are you?

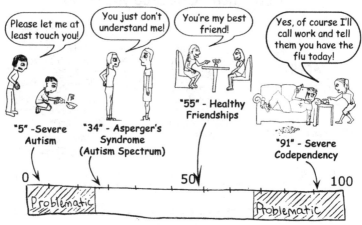

Degree of Connectedness to Others

Neurotic vs. Obnoxious:
"How much BLAME do you cast?"

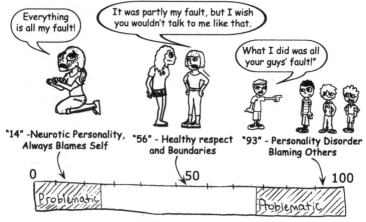

Amount of Blame Cast to Others

SECTION II

THE 8 PRIMARY SPECTRUMS OF PSYCHIATRY

CHAPTER 6

THE DEPRESSION SPECTRUM: SHALLOWNESS VS. DESPAIR

DEPRESSION-WHAT'S NEW IN DSM-5 AND DSM-5-TR?

The concept of chronicity in *Depressive Disorders* changes in DSM-5 and DSM-5-TR. *Dysthymia*, a smoldering, mild to moderate depression that presumably never meets the criteria for *Major Depression* and lasts at least two years, has been eliminated. In its place is the diagnosis of **Persistent Depressive Disorder**, which now encompasses chronic *Major Depression* as well as *Dysthymic Disorder*.

The distinguishing feature in DSM-5-TR (and DSM-5) is the chronic, *Persistent* nature of the mood disturbance. The degree of severity is deemphasized and, in its place, the degree of persistence is given priority. This is consistent with the common clinical presentation of recurring mood disorders. Severity often fluctuates dramatically, but the persistence of melancholy remains a hallmark. Clinicians are permitted to include all the variations and tones of depressed mood when diagnosing *Persistent Depressive Disorder*, provided they demonstrate the feature of *persistence*.

In addition, clinicians may utilize the *Mixed features specifiers* to document depression with significant *bipolarity*. Similarly, clinicians can document the presence of anxiety associated with depression by using the *Anxiety specifiers*. DSM-5-TR, like DSM-5, no longer treats bereavement as an exclusionary criterion for the diagnosis of depression. Actively grieving patients can also be diagnosed with depression.

 Furthermore, two new diagnoses were added to the depression category in DSM-5 (and continued in DSM-5-TR), namely, **Premenstrual Dysphoric Disorder (PMDD)** and **Disruptive Mood Dysregulation Disorder**. Controversy has surrounded *Premenstrual Dysphoric Disorder* for years. In 1914, Lita Stetter Hollingsworth sought to establish that women were not impaired as a result of their menstrual cycles.[13] The controversy around this disorder unfortunately continues.[14] Differentiating between *PMDD* from other serious psychiatric conditions like *Bipolar Disorder* has important implications for treatment.[15]

Premenstrual Dysphoric Disorder involves depressive symptoms in women occurring in the final week before onset of menses with improvement beginning shortly after menses begins. The remainder of the menstrual cycle is either free of symptoms or symptoms are minimal.

Disruptive Mood Dysregulation Disorder (Must be evidenced between ages 6 and 10) is characterized by severe and persistent irritability. This new diagnostic category involves frequent outbursts combined with a persistent angry/irritable backdrop. Onset must be prior to age 10 years.

DSM-5-TR saw the addition of a new depressive diagnosis, namely **Prolonged Grief Disorder**. It pertains to intense yearning or preoccupation of the deceased loved one beyond one year from their death. Three or more emotional symptoms are required as well. One-in-10 adults are at risk for developing *Prolonged Grief Disorder* after the death of a loved one.

THE DEPRESSION SPECTRUM: SHALLOWNESS VS. DESPAIR

 DSM-5-TR restored *Unspecified Mood Disorder,* a diagnosis that had been removed from the prior DSM edition. Its elimination had proven problematic for some clinicians when presenting mood symptoms failed to fit clearly with depression or bipolar criteria. *Unspecified Mood Disorder* allows the diagnosis to maintain a level of uncertainty, while still documenting the presence of mood symptoms.

 DSM-5-TR also added symptom codes for *suicidal behavior* and *nonsuicidal self-injury.*

DEPRESSION AS A SPECTRUM OF ILLNESS

DSM-5's introduction of the concept of illness along a spectrum abandoned the binary, black-and-white distinctions of DSM-IV in favor of a gradation of functioning and severity of presentation.

Shallowness vs. Despair
"How much SORROW do you hold?"

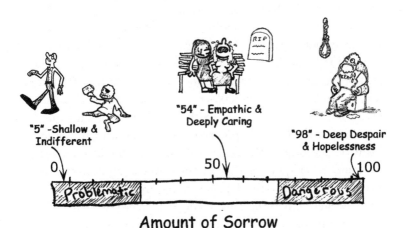

Amount of Sorrow

A certain degree of sadness and depression is part of everyday life and can be considered normal when viewed from the perspective of depression along a spectrum.

Shallow, indifferent individuals who may seem immune from sad emotion tend to engage in limited or almost no introspection. Such people might have difficulty learning from their mistakes and may be less prone to sorrowful emotions.

In contrast, the deeply despairing person tends to engage in endless brooding and introspection. Such individuals may mull things over to such exaggerated degrees that they become paralyzed and feel crushed by their ceaseless ruminations and regurgitations of the past. Toward the middle of this spectrum, an individual experiences sorrow, depth of emotion, and a reasonable degree of interiority without undue, fruitless suffering. Sorrow and regret may be critical to character formation and the cultivation of empathy and the capacity for self-reflection. Rumi, the mystic poet wrote, "The wound is the place where the light enters you."

CASE EXAMPLE

Richard, a compilation of various patients who might be located on the lower end of this scale, presents for treatment at the insistence of his spouse. Richard's wife describes him as aloof and distant, unable to relate to her emotions. Richard has been successful in his career but has few friends. If he has regrets and sorrows, he gives little or no indication. Richard suffers from a conspicuous lack of introspection, and if he does think about himself and his life, it tends to appear shallow and inconsequential. This lack of capacity for sorrow along with the absence of introspection interferes with Richard's ability to empathize with his children, his wife, and others. Richard has been to marital counseling, but he could never quite grasp that there was anything wrong. For Richard, life is all right. Upon entering treatment, Richard may acknowledge something must change only because someone else, like his wife, made this clear to him. Any recognition of the need for treatment is not the result of interior reflection.

Richard's work in therapy may require him to cultivate the capacity to feel sorrow, discontent, and introspection. Richard may never become warm and fuzzy; however, he can develop sufficient tolerance for sorrow and introspection to equip him to empathize with his wife and others.

Of course, it is far more likely that persons located closer to 100 on this scale will present for treatment. These individuals often suffer deep depression, characterized by a lack of energy, hopelessness, and despair. Their condition can become so profound as to cause them to contemplate suicide. Clinicians will find themselves working diligently to help such individuals move closer to the middle range where they diminish the severe, relentless self-examination and condemnation. Treatment may not achieve a *Confucian* ideal of the middle way, however, and some individuals will continue to suffer lingering, persistent depressive symptoms.

CONFUCIAN DOCTRINE OF THE MEAN

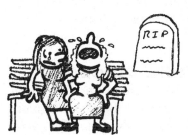

To find oneself in the middle range is optimal. The middle domain allows a person to profit and gain something from losses and regrets without becoming overwhelmed by them. Empathy, insight, improved self-regulation, and the fruits of explorative psychotherapy arise from this region. There is a fluidity that characterizes the middle range that allows a person to descend into the darker realms of human existence while preserving the capacity to emerge again into an engaged, active life. Not only are sorrow and introspection tolerated in the middle region, but they can also be transmuted into useful results that help forge a person's character. In the middle, life experience is like humus in the topsoil that is turned, worked, and eventually provides the required nutrients for soul building. In the middle region, people do not need to resort to aloof disengagement, nor do they need to fear becoming engulfed by their own despair.

MAJOR DEPRESSIVE DISORDER... "SIG E CAPSS" FOR AT LEAST 2 WEEKS

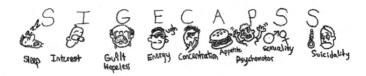

Major Depressive Disorder is a very common complaint that leads people to seek treatment. Severe cases of *Major Depressive Disorder* are challenging to treat. Many clinicians have received the middle-of-the-night call from people declaring they want to die. Depression is one of the deepest forms of human sufferings, and suicide or thoughts of suicide are among its hallmark features.

The diagnosis of *Major Depressive Disorder* is established by a constellation of symptoms that must be present for a sufficient duration. While it technically only requires two weeks of symptoms, most patients who present for treatment have suffered for months or years. Treatment typically includes psychotherapy, antidepressant medications, or combinations of both.

PERSISTENT DEPRESSIVE DISORDER

Persistent Depressive Disorder consolidates *Major Depression, Recurrent* (or *Chronic*) and *Dysthymic Disorder*. Based on diagnostic
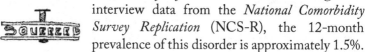
interview data from the *National Comorbidity Survey Replication* (NCS-R), the 12-month prevalence of this disorder is approximately 1.5%. The causes of *Persistent Depressive Disorder* are complex and can include genetic factors, substance abuse, stress, interpersonal issues, endocrinologic factors, childhood issues, trauma, and more. These complex factors make *Persistent Depressive Disorder* difficult to treat. Treatment inevitably involves the simultaneous use of several different approaches.

PREMENSTRUAL DYSPHORIC DISORDER

Some women experience physical and emotional symptoms prior to the onset of menstruation. These symptoms range in severity from mild, barely noticeable changes, to severe, disruptive changes. Mood symptoms can include severe mood swings, irritability, anger outbursts, anxiety, and severe depression. Symptoms resolve or substantially improve once menstruation ensues. Women with significant complaints may be diagnosed with *Premenstrual Dysphoric Disorder*. Their lives are shackled to their monthly cycle in ways that can have serious adverse impacts. Treatments for *Premenstrual Dysphoric Disorder* include exercise, diet, antidepressant medication, antianxiety medication, hormonal treatment, and psychotherapy.

CONCLUSION

Depressive disorders are common and produce substantial suffering and economic burden.[16] Familiarity with how to diagnose and treat them is a critically important task for any mental health care provider.

CHAPTER 7

THE MANIA SPECTRUM: BORING VS. BIPOLAR

BIPOLAR—WHAT'S NEW IN DSM-5-TR

The core criteria for **Bipolar Disorder** give more emphasis to increased energy and increased activity levels than on the qualities of mood. Just as with *Depressive Disorder*, the clinician can specify the presence of *Mixed Features* when significant depressive symptoms exist and *Anxiety* when there is an anxious component. According to Jules Angst, "a weakness, shown in relation to DSM-IV, was *that it was only able to formally diagnose under half the patients actually treated.*[17]

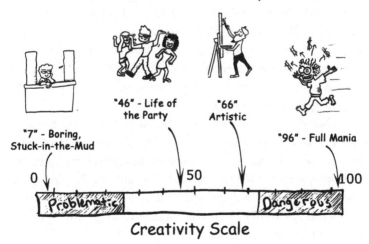

Boring vs. Bipolar
"How much CREATIVITY do you have?"

Creativity Scale

BIPOLAR AS A SPECTRUM OF ILLNESS

In the last decade, *Bipolar Disorder* received a great deal of attention. There are suggestions that it has become a "trend" to diagnose *Bipolar Disorder* in virtually all circumstances where mood and affect instability exists. Clinicians may even have encountered patients who come seeking a diagnosis of *Bipolar Disorder*. Angst criticized earlier versions of the DSM for "... the lack of operationalized subthreshold diagnoses."[18] The rise in the rate of diagnosis differs between adults and youths. According to one study, "While the diagnosis of bipolar disorder in adults increased nearly 2-fold during a 10-year study period, the diagnosis of bipolar disorder in youth increased approximately 40-fold during this period."[19] The reasons for the rise in rates of diagnosis or the reason for the discrepancies between adults and youth are unclear. Perhaps greater media attention combined with the barrage of advertising from pharmaceutical companies that see enormous potential in treating unstable mood and affect contributed to this. *Disruptive Mood Disorder* served to reduce the overdiagnosis of *Bipolar Disorder* in children who displayed persistent irritability with temper outbursts without other symptoms of mania.

Patients who present with a full array of bipolar symptoms that include discrete episodes of mania and depression are easily diagnosed. Because full-blown mania often leads to prompt hospitalization, many clinicians may have little experience with true mania. Muted presentations of *Bipolar Disorder* are likely to be more familiar. Clinicians may need to rely on symptoms that are strongly suggestive of *Bipolar Disorder*.

When the diagnosis is unclear, heavier reliance on a history of bipolarity or evaluation of "how much" bipolarity a person displays may be useful indicators. Such approaches reflect the spirit of a *spectrum approach* to *Bipolar Disorder*. Recognizing *Bipolarity*, even when all the required diagnostic criteria for *Bipolar Disorder* are not met, helps codify important clinical findings and may have important treatment implications.

THE MANIA SPECTRUM: BORING VS. BIPOLAR 49

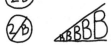

The concept of "how much" bipolarity exists can be reassuring, even liberating for many patients. Imagine that all of us exist along a continuum of bipolarity somewhere between "0" bipolarity and "100" bipolarity. Either extreme of the spectrum typically proves to be problematic.

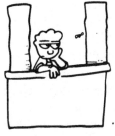

Toward the low end of the spectrum, toward "zero," a person possesses very low energy. Such a person tends to lack creativity and may be perceived as boring or flat. Such a person is caricatured as being stuck in an office cubicle, surrounded by stacks of paper, partaking in no creative outlets in their job or elsewhere. There is a pronounced absence of *joie de vivre* (exuberant enjoyment of life). Such a person suffers a global lack of energy and motivation. The person's life may appear dull, lacking in spontaneity, and chorelike. This person desperately needs more life force, more *Eros*, and more spontaneity.

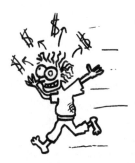

At the other end of the spectrum (toward "100"), different problems ensue. Such individuals suffer an overabundance of energy. They cannot slow down, they tend to be too talkative, they become flooded with ideas, their thoughts race, and they may experience frank psychosis with hallucinations. Frequently, they overspend with a lack of restraint or good judgment. They may give away their possessions. Their speech is impulsive and tends to be unfiltered. Those situated toward "100" on the spectrum will often take risks that others judge to be excessive; they display poor judgment in various matters. Such symptoms need urgent treatment.

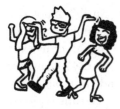

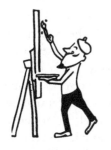

Most of us are somewhere in between these two extremes. At various times, we may tend toward less energy and less spontaneity, or we may lean toward higher energy and creativity. Toward the middle of the spectrum there is a wide range that encompasses healthy human behavior. The cartoon image in this middle area depicts someone dancing, painting, and enjoying life. The person may be fun, "cool," and the "life of the party." Further up the scale, a person shows signs of gifted artistry. Those at the lower end of the scale might not be the life of the party, but neither are they a black hole of lethargy. *Bipolarity* that remains at sustainable levels, without extremes in either direction, is a blessing. A wellspring of creative, artistic energy can be tapped without demonstrating disruptive extremes. This degree of *Bipolarity* is modulated such that a person is equipped to engage life, engage with others, create from nothing, and experience excitement about living. Treatment may need to be considered when there exists far too much or utter absence of *bipolarity*.

CLINICAL EXAMPLE

Gloria presented for treatment when things had gone too far. She had always been a fun-loving, gregarious person who enjoyed going out with friends. She worked as an interior designer at a well-known firm, where she had been one of the best at her work. When life became more stressful than usual, her sleep worsened. She regretted a series of bad investments; she became more irritable; and she became more easily distracted. She had become impulsive. She had been counseled at work for blurting out things that came to her mind. Her spending habits had been out of control for months, and her drinking escalated. Gloria had been in a monogamous relationship for several years but recently had a one-night stand with someone she met while out of town.

The straw that broke the camel's back was when she screamed obscenities at her boss, a man she had always admired. While Gloria displayed no psychosis, she certainly had many symptoms along the spectrum of *Bipolarity*. Clearly, her extreme mood was causing problems.

With the help of mood-stabilizing medication, something to improve her sleep, and counseling, Gloria accepted the idea that treatment could modify and even subdue some of her symptoms without entirely ridding her of all her *Bipolarity*. Instead, the goal became a manageable state of creativity and excitement. This honored her creativity while recognizing the need for moderation. As her insomnia, irritability, and impulsivity calmed down, she recovered the ability to "govern" herself and manage her extremes.

CONCLUSION

Bipolar and Related Disorders are common conditions encountered by mental health practitioners. Discussing *Bipolarity* as a *Spectrum* can help patients embrace treatment while preserving their dignity and respect. Even in situations where the boundary between normal creativity and pathology is unclear, the spectrum between *Boring* and *Bipolar* can be a useful construct.

CHAPTER 8

THE ANXIETY SPECTRUM: CARELESSNESS VS. ANXIOUSNESS

ANXIETY—WHAT'S NEW IN DSM-5/TR

Starting in DSM-5, several diagnoses were no longer found in the *Anxiety Disorder* section.

Obsessive Compulsive and Related Disorders comprised a new category, and OCD was relocated under this heading.

PTSD moved under the heading of *Trauma- and Stressor-Related Disorders*. The *Anxiety Disorder* section also uncoupled the diagnoses of *Panic* and *Agoraphobia*.

Separation Anxiety Disorder and *Selective Mutism* moved from the *Disorders of Childhood* section to the *Anxiety Disorder* section.

ANXIETY AS A SPECTRUM OF ILLNESS

When considering *Anxiety Disorders* along a spectrum, the amount of *vigilance* is the fulcrum on which these phenomena pivot. Extremes of *Carelessness* versus *Anxiousness* characterize this spectrum.

53

Carelessness vs. Anxiousness
"How much VIGILANCE do you have?"

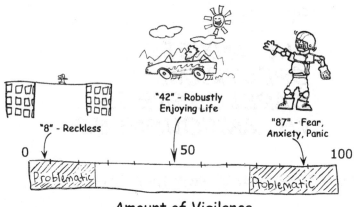

Here the question becomes "How much vigilance do you have?" The more vigilance people display, the more likely they are to progress to clinical anxiety at some point.

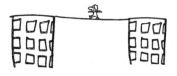

The far-left side of the spectrum involves almost no vigilance at all. Carelessness can be highly problematic. Such a person may behave recklessly with an inability to properly evaluate risk. Anxiety is a warning system for our body and mind that something dangerous may be at hand. The capacity to arouse the autonomic nervous system to elicit the *fight-or-flight* response is vitally important. According to *Kaplan & Saddock: Concise Guide to Psychiatry*:

> An important aspect of emotions is their effect on the selectivity of attention. Anxious persons likely select certain things in their environment and overlook others in their effort to prove that they are justified in considering the situation frightening. If they falsely justify their fear, they augment their anxieties by the selective response and set up a

vicious circle of anxiety, distorted perception, and increased anxiety. If, alternatively, they falsely reassure themselves by selective thinking, appropriate anxiety may be reduced, and they may fail to take necessary precautions.[20]

Vigilance is necessary to avoid danger. Depicted in the cartoon at the left side of the scale is a tightrope walker with no net, showing very little vigilance and considerable recklessness.

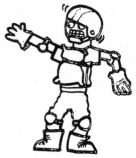

The other end of the spectrum depicts someone possessed of too much vigilance. This person is highly anxious and fearful. The figure is covered with protective gear, including a helmet, gloves, boots, kneepads, and even a pillow strapped to his chest to protect him from falls and other dangers. This is someone who is too cautious, too anxious, and too easily overwhelmed by fear. Such people may have *Panic Disorder*, *Generalized Anxiety Disorder*, or another anxiety-related illness. Such a high degree of hypervigilance interferes with life.

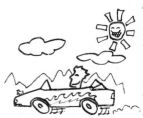

The well-balanced person is depicted as riding down the road in a convertible with the top down. The sun is shining, and though the person is driving carefully, care and caution are not hindering enjoyment. The person balances the risk of driving with the top down with the pleasure of driving a convertible. Such people have found themselves in the sweet spot between appropriate concern or worry and a lack of hypervigilance that would rob life of lightness of being.

PANIC DISORDER

Panic Disorder manifests with very intense anxiety that can be terrifying to patients. The initial episode of panic is frequently remembered in vivid detail. *Panic Disorder* is composed of discrete episodes of *panic anxiety* and frequently includes *anticipatory anxiety*. During acute bouts of panic, patients may be afraid they are having a heart attack or that they are going to die. A host of physical symptoms may occur during a panic episode. Patients may present repeatedly to their physician or to an emergency department for evaluation of various symptoms associated with panic anxiety. After extensive testing fails to determine a clear cause, *Panic Disorder* may be diagnosed by default. This is often the precipitant for a referral to a mental health professional. Cognitive behavioral psychotherapy combined with low-dose antidepressants are common treatment strategies. Brief courses of antianxiety agents, often administered under the tongue for faster onset of action, can help restore a sense of control to patients, but whenever possible, caution should be exercised in using antianxiety agents like benzodiazepines (e.g., Alprazolam and Lorazepam) in patients with *Panic Disorder*. Though the controversies surrounding long-term use of benzodiazepine are not resolved, the bias against their use has been questioned.[21]

GENERALIZED ANXIETY DISORDER (GAD)

The person with *GAD* is a worrier. Such persons worry about money, health, stress, work, home, play, and anything else they can imagine. Physical symptoms such as tension, fatigue, poor concentration, insomnia, and irritability frequently accompany their chronic worry and anxiety. While *GAD* appears less acute and less overwhelming than *Panic Disorder*, it produces considerable distress. Treatment may involve psychotherapy, biofeedback, antidepressant medications, beta blockers, and occasional sparing use of sedatives.

SOCIAL ANXIETY (PHOBIA)

The lifetime prevalence of *Social Phobia* is approximately 4%.[22] It seems to occur in people who are also shy and introverted. Sufferers hate being in the spotlight or drawing attention to themselves. Interacting with strangers can be exquisitely painful. Their numerous anxieties cause the sufferer to avoid anxiety-provoking situations. This disorder can be debilitating, and sufferers often limit their social, educational, and career opportunities because of their pervasive anxiety. Treatment involves psychotherapy, skills training, antidepressants, and occasionally sedatives. Validation of the specific features of *Social Phobia* goes a long way to easing the alienation felt by its sufferers.

SPECIFIC PHOBIA

Specific Phobias include a broad range of fears that arise in relation to a specific stimulus. Common phobias include fear of heights, fear of snakes, and fear of spiders. Because the provocation can be very circumscribed, avoidance is most likely to prove effective. When exposure to the stimulus cannot be avoided or if the symptoms severely interfere with functioning, patients may seek treatment. *Cognitive Behavior Therapy* can be very helpful in reducing specific fears. *Systematic Desensitization,* as well as *Flooding* techniques, can also prove helpful.

CONCLUSION

Anxiety symptoms are very common in the general population. They are frequently seen in combination with other illnesses such as *Major Depressive Disorder.* Anxiety has adaptive and maladaptive aspects. One way of conceptualizing *Anxiety Disorders* is to imagine the symptoms pivoting around the axis of vigilance.

CHAPTER 9

THE PSYCHOSIS SPECTRUM: VISIONLESS VERSUS PSYCHOTIC

WHAT'S NEW IN DSM-5 / DSM-5-TR

The five subtypes of *Schizophrenia* have been eliminated (catatonic, disorganized, paranoid, residual, and undifferentiated). *Catatonia*, however, is still used as a specifier that can be employed with *Schizophrenia, Bipolar Disorder* or *Depression*. The diagnoses of schizophrenia must now include at least one positive symptom—hallucinations, delusions, or disorganized speech.

With *Schizoaffective Disorder*, either depression or bipolarity must be present for most of the disorder's total duration.

PSYCHOSIS AS A SPECTRUM OF ILLNESSES

Of the *8 Primary Spectrums of Psychiatry* described in this book that exist along a continuum between normal functioning and illness, psychosis is the hardest one in which to identify a range of normal expression. Is there really any degree to which psychosis can be construed as falling within the range of normal human experience? If we change "how psychotic are you?" to "how strong are your dreams and visions?" a spectrum begins to emerge for the cluster of symptoms common to psychosis. Almost everyone has some level of inspiring dreams or visions. We may awaken in the middle of the night convinced that something has happened and be surprised to realize it was "just a dream." For those few minutes in which we are out of touch with reality, we are still possessed by the dream. Sometimes the breakthrough of an unusually inspiring thought or idea can radically alter our perspective on reality. Such occurrences might seem to come from outside oneself. Many people have heard voices, seen things that others did not see, or experienced moments of precognition. Strictly speaking, these may be considered hallucinations or delusions. They can also be considered as eruptions from other parts of the psyche, perhaps even beyond the psyche. Poets, authors, and artists sometimes describe "being a channel for the art trying to incarnate itself." They claim that they didn't produce it themselves but were merely vessels of transmission. Others will have powerful spiritual experiences. They may see a vision of a deceased relative, hear their voice briefly, or even be convinced they hear God speak to them at times. Such unconventional views could easily be construed as distorted and bordering on delusional by someone else. This may not signify formal psychosis but instead may be a feature of normal human experience of the divine or the normal grieving process after the loss of a loved one. One common feature is that they lie along a spectrum of various intensities of dreams and visions. If these dreams and visions become intense and overwhelming

Visionless vs. Psychotic:
"How strong are your DREAMS and VISIONS?"

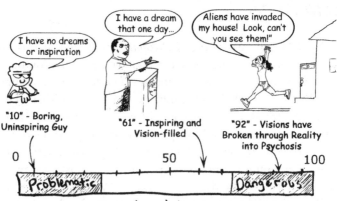

Intensity of Dreams and Visions

enough, a breakdown between real and unreal can occur. A vision or voice can persist and be so intense or bizarre that there would be a consensus that it is abnormal. But we propose that even psychosis covers a domain that includes "normal" human experience.

Our illustration is titled *"Visionless vs. Psychotic: How strong are your dreams and visions?"* The scale on the bottom indicates the strength of these dreams and visions. As usual, either end of the spectrum is problematic, and trying to hold fast to the middle yields the optimal results.

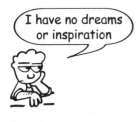

On the left end of the spectrum is an individual with no dreams or inspirations. They are a boring sort, with little spontaneity or future goals. It's hard for them to imagine life in the future since their imagination is so limited. They had trouble playing any games as a child that required thinking outside the box, role-playing, or other imaginal pieces. When they tried to draw a picture, their mind and imagination were empty and the paper remained blank. They disliked art, drama, or even theoretical physics in college; they required too much imagination. Spirituality and metaphysics do not attract them, since they have difficulty seeing anything beyond the physical reality of the here and now. They cannot remember any of their dreams and do not experience inspiring thoughts. They may have a hard time making career choices or choosing where to live because they are devoid of vision for the future. While such a person doesn't always come in for treatment, this individual deeply needs the help of a skilled psychotherapist or a spiritual director to get them out of this dry, lifeless space.

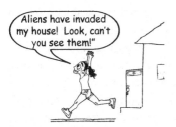

The person on the right has a different and more serious problem. Such people are being flooded by the dream world, and their imagination is no longer in touch with reality. They have lost the filter that most of us possess, that allows us to know the difference between what is real and what is fantasy. They are full of delusions and they have become convinced that aliens have invaded our planet and are taking over their neighborhood.

They have visual hallucinations, seeing images of these aliens attacking. They further believe someone has been monitoring their phone and spying on their actions. They hear voices incessantly. The voices give them instructions, as if to direct their thoughts and actions. The voices are sometimes dark and critical and occasionally tell them to give up or take their own life. These sorts of psychotic symptoms can be terrifying. It is arguably the most severe of our psychiatric diagnoses. Such a person is in urgent need of hospitalization, antipsychotic medications, and acute stabilization.

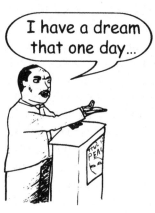

As always, the middle region of the spectrum is the optimal realm. This is where the soul thrives and where we can reach our highest potential. It is the land of the visionaries that we all admire or strive to become and where occasionally we all dwell. It is the domain that gives rise to people like Martin Luther King Jr., Mother Teresa, Mahatma Gandhi, John F. Kennedy, and countless others who inspire us. People living in the middle of this spectrum are full of inspirations, hopes, and dreams.

Most people have visionary moments in their life, in which they are swept up in something larger than themselves. Perhaps you have awakened in the middle of the night, awestruck with a new idea and the possibilities it offers. On such occasions, you have entered the middle region between boring and psychotic. Such moments need not be grand, sometimes they may involve the solution to a vexing problem or the unexpected reminder of a special occasion of a loved one. Any powerful new idea, goal, vision, or hope may be found in this territory. Whereas psychosis can be a terrifying experience that threatens to rupture our psychological container, experiences arising in the middle region of this spectrum can be profound and transformative, catalyzing enormous change. At times, the experience of being comfortably in this middle region is rich, meaningful, and even sacramental. Life is neither bland nor excessively spicy; it has the right seasoning to bring out the best flavor.

DIAGNOSES IN DETAIL

SCHIZOPHRENIA

Schizophrenia involves losing touch with reality. It often includes hallucinations that are defined by a perception without an associated stimulus. They include auditory, visual, tactile, and/or olfactory hallucinations. Persons with schizophrenia can be disorganized and act in highly unusual ways. Delusions, defined as fixed, false beliefs, are often present and can be bizarre at times.

SCHIZOAFFECTIVE DISORDER

Schizoaffective Disorder is best thought of as a mixture of symptoms and signs that are associated with *Schizophrenia* and mood disorders (bipolar or depression). Individuals with *Schizoaffective Disorder* must have evidence of a major mood disorder present the majority of the time that they are symptomatic. Like *Schizophrenia*, this disorder can be quite debilitating.

Delusional Disorder is characterized by a well-circumscribed delusion in the context of otherwise well-preserved functioning.

CONCLUSION

Psychosis viewed along a spectrum spans a terrifying realm of human experience, as well as the realm from which inspiration and visionary ideas arise. Clinicians do well to remember that there is often a fine line that separates madness and genius. The middle region of the *Psychosis Spectrum* is fertile and inspired. It does not lead others to immediately conclude that a person is insane. By viewing psychosis along a spectrum from thoroughly boring and uninspired to fully overtaken by visions and delusions, the clinician can navigate the inner landscape with a proper balance of re spect, caution, and inspiration of their own.

CHAPTER 10

THE FOCUS SPECTRUM: ATTENTION DEFICIT DISORDER VS. OBSESSIVE COMPULSIVE DISORDERS

ADHD AND OCD—WHAT'S NEW IN DSM-5/TR

DSM-5 added a new group of disorders known as the *Obsessive Compulsive and Related Disorders*. This category includes *Obsessive Compulsive Disorder (OCD)*, *Body Dysmorphic Disorder*, and *Trichotillomania*.

There are newly created diagnoses in this section that include *Hoarding Disorder* and *Excoriation (skin picking) Disorder*.

Attention Deficit Hyperactivity Disorder (ADHD) has remained virtually unchanged.

ADHD AND OCD AS A SPECTRUM

The spectrum proposed here combines two categories in DSM-5-TR that can be related to one another by the degree of sustained focus a person maintains. Strictly speaking, *OCD's* ancestral roots link it to anxiety disorders and not *ADHD*. However, these two disorders move about an axis that is related to how much capacity for focused attention the patient displays. Someone with very

65

little focus might be suffering from *Attention Deficit Hyperactivity Disorder*, while somebody with extreme focus, perhaps even an inability to change their focus of attention from a ruminative thought, might be diagnosed with *Obsessive Compulsive Disorder*.

Attention Deficit Disorder (ADHD) vs. Obsessive Compulsive Disorder (OCD)
"How much FOCUS do you have?"

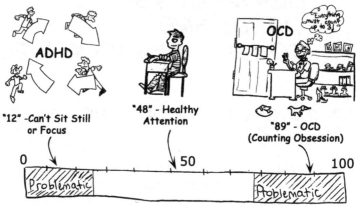

Amount of Focusing Ability

In our illustration, we have labeled the primary, determinant variable as the amount of focusing someone tends to display.

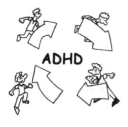

The far left of the diagram depicts a person with almost no focusing ability. Such people cannot maintain focus on a single task for very long. Their mind wanders; they are very distractible and jump from project to project. This person is depicted as having *ADHD*.

Equally problematic is the other end of the spectrum on the right side of the diagram. Such people have too much focus. They are unable to shift their focus of attention and often go over the same detail or worry repeatedly. Persons with *OCD* become locked

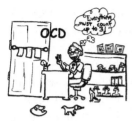

into obsessive patterns of thinking. These patterns may include counting rituals, hand-washing, excessive orderliness, a need for symmetry, germ phobias, and a myriad of other obsessions. The consequences of such ceaseless obsessions, compulsions, and rituals range from mild annoyance to significant impairment in work and social life. Severely afflicted individuals appear to be enslaved by their obsessive-compulsive rituals and routines. Treatment often consists of medications (most commonly SSRIs) and behavioral treatment.

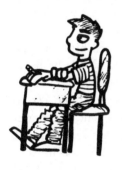

The middle part of the diagram depicts the area of healthy focus. Here, a person is shown whose degree of focus is properly balanced. Such individuals can pay attention for extended periods of time, for example, in a lecture. Their ability to maintain their focus of attention still allows for flexible shifts in attention. They are not imprisoned by their attention, like someone with *OCD*, but can flexibly allow their thoughts and actions to shift from one focus to another. People located in the middle region of this spectrum will not drift aimlessly or haphazardly from one topic to another, nor will they gravitate to every shiny new object they encounter, as the person with *ADHD* might do. Individuals with *ADHD* have difficulty sustaining attention when something ceases to be of high interest to them. The ideal or goal with regard to the *Focus Spectrum* is to strike an effective balance between a well-focused attention and a shifting focus of attention. This is the middle ground. Straying to either extreme end of the spectrum proves problematic and often requires *professional* attention.

CLINICAL EXAMPLE

Pete is a patient whose focus places him at the extreme end. He has always been an orderly and high-achieving man. As a child,

Pete kept his room neat and clean, he turned in his homework on time after checking it over numerous times, and he often felt anxious that he might have done something wrong that would come back to haunt him. He excelled in school and was well-liked. Pete's tendencies and idiosyncrasies intensified when he reached high school. He would become terribly upset and anxious if his homework was not exactly right, and this required him to spend long hours completing assignments, longer than others thought necessary. His morning routine to get ready for school took progressively longer as he added more rituals that had to be performed in the exact same way and in the same order each day. Upon graduation from high school, Pete took a job overseeing quality control at a local factory. His relentless attention to detail garnered favorable attention at work, though many coworkers, who found his perfectionism unbearable, disliked him. He kept both his home and workplace spotlessly clean. When he began to feel that there were germs on various surfaces, he started using *Clorox* wipes on his phone, keyboard, countertops, and certain personal belongings. By the time he sought treatment, he reported that he was cleaning the kitchen four times a day, he had rituals that governed how his dishes should be stacked, and was insistent that toilet paper rolls be hung a certain way (over the top). Pete's friends poked fun at him for his overly focused attention by sometimes leaving small pieces of trash on the floor to see how long it would take him to notice and clean it up.

A year before he sought treatment, Pete's mother was diagnosed with emphysema that required her to rely on continuous oxygen. One day the idea popped into his head that she might run out of oxygen, so he began calling her five times a day to make sure her breathing was all right. He found it hard to fall asleep, as he began to worry before bed about her health. His focus on germs increased and he began washing his hands every 20 or 30 minutes. His hands became red and excoriated. He developed beliefs, in which he grew convinced that if he did not pray in a certain manner and at certain times, God would not hear his prayers and his mother might die. If he messed up one word in the prayer, he felt compelled to start from the beginning and pray again. The numerous things he felt the need to focus upon, consumed more time, and Pete began to withdraw from people. When the COVID-19 pandemic appeared, Pete's hand-washing was out of control.

He was referred for treatment when his hand-washing resulted in severe dermatitis. He was diagnosed with OCD, started on a serotonergic anti- depressant (sertraline, *Zoloft*), and referred for *Cognitive Behavioral Therapy*. The medicine helped Pete loosen his focus of attention on the things that now were plaguing him, and psychotherapy helped reduce his exaggerated focus as well. Pete learned to redirect his focus of attention away from obsessive ruminations, and with the help of the medicine, he found he could free himself from the endless loops and eddies of thought he had known his entire life. Pete was pleased to discover that medicine and therapy did nothing to loosen his careful attention to detail at work, but he no longer felt compelled to correct coworkers' every mistake, just the ones that affected quality control.

DIAGNOSES IN DETAIL

OBSESSIVE COMPULSIVE DISORDER AND RELATED DISORDERS

The *Obsessive Compulsive and Related Disorders* are grouped in a distinct place from *ADHD* in DSM-5-TR. Clinicians should keep in mind that the *Focus Spectrum* provides a model for understanding a *spectrum* concept and is not intended to conflate the diagnoses of *ADHD* and *OCD*.

OCD and related disorders have in common an excessive degree of focus. These disorders include:

Obsessive Compulsive Disorder (OCD) is characterized by *Obsessions* that consist of persistent, intrusive, unwanted thoughts, urges, or images and *Compulsions* that are repetitive behaviors intended to suppress or neutralize obsessions with other thoughts or actions. Both obsessions and compulsions are time-consuming and distressing.

Common symptoms include rituals involving checking, counting, cleaning, and the need for symmetry. Sufferers may have fears of losing con trol or may worry incessantly that they will engage in forbidden actions. Clinicians can specify the degree of insight (good, fair, and poor). There is also a *tic-related specifier* available. Even those with insight are often unable to fend off their OCD symptoms. Treatment may include medications and cognitive behavioral psychotherapy. Medications are most often serotonergic antidepressants, usually at higher dosages.

Body Dysmorphic Disorder can be a very challenging illness to treat. Patients become utterly convinced that they have a severe body defect, usually cosmetic in nature. Even if there is a slight defect, their obsession about this small defect is much greater than is warranted. They overly focus on their perceived defect. They may consult plastic surgeons who hesitate to operate when their perceived defect is not detectable or objectively verified.[23] At some point in the disorder, sufferers will have engaged in repetitive checking behaviors. Medications can help slightly, but often response is marginal. Psychotherapy is the most effective course, and cognitive behavioral therapy, consisting of elements such as exposure, response prevention, behavioral experiments, and cognitive restructuring, is perhaps the most common type of psychotherapy employed.

Trichotillomania presents with recurrent hair pulling resulting in hair loss. There is a cycle of tension (when hair pulling is resisted) and relief (when hair pulling ensues). These features produce significant distress and impairment.

Hoarding Disorder involves the inability to discard possessions, regardless of their value (or lack of value). Sufferers perceive the need to save things and become distressed when having to discard them. The person with *Hoarding Disorder* often suffers great distress and impairment.

Excoriation (skin picking) Disorder manifests with skin picking that results in lesions or skin infections. The common features of tension and relief found in trichotillomania, and the elements of distress and impairment are characteristic.

ADHD (NEURODEVELOMENTAL DISORDERS)

Attention Deficit Hyperactivity Disorder (ADHD) includes two broad symptom clusters, *Inattention* and *Hyperactivity/Impulsivity*. The disorder re sults in social, occupational, or school impairment.

ADHD is usually diagnosed in childhood. School-aged children may demonstrate difficulty in the classroom deriving their inattention and/or hy peractivity. Work may be left unfinished, homework may not be turned in, disruptive behavior may occur in the classroom. The hyperactive compo nents may include restlessness, fidgetiness, calling out in class, and other inappropriate behavior. While *ADHD* may improve by adulthood, the symptoms often persist causing difficulties in work and personal life.[24][25][26][27] A multimodal treatment that includes behavior modification, medica tions, or combinations of the two is common.[28] Various medications are used including stimulants (amphetamine and amphetamine-like medications), antidepressants, atomoxetine *(Strattera,* a nonstimulant, norepinephrine reuptake inhibitor), antihypertensive agents (adrenergic agonists like clonidine, *Catapres,* or guanfacine hydrochloride, *Tenex).* Close coordination with teachers and the education of families are crucial.

CONCLUSION

Although DSM-5-TR does not in any way link *ADHD* and *OCD*, a common thread courses through them both. The amount of focus a person displays can be a defining feature of where a person lies on this spectrum. For persons at the left end of this spectrum (*ADHD*), treatment strives to in crease their ability to sustain their focus of attention. For persons at the right end of the spectrum (*OCD*), the goal is to temper their excessive focus of attention.

CHAPTER 11

THE SUBSTANCE ABUSE SPECTRUM: ASCETIC VS. ADDICTED

"It is impossible to understand addiction without asking what relief the addict finds, or hopes to find, in the drug or the addictive behaviour."
(Excerpt from *In the Realm of Hungry Ghosts* by Gabor Matte)

SUBSTANCE-RELATED AND ADDICTIVE DISORDERS—WHAT'S NEW IN DSM-5/TR

There are several changes in DSM-5 and DSM-5-TR pertaining to substance abuse.

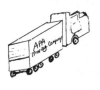

Gambling Disorder is now recognized as sharing so many features with substance abuse disorders that it was moved to this category. One big change occurring with DSM-5 was that no longer was a distinction made between *substance abuse* and *substance dependence*. DSM-5 and DSM-5-TR adopt a "spectrum" approach. *Substance-related and Addictive Disorders* encompass *Alcohol-related Disorder, Cannabis-related Disorder, Opioid-related Disorder, Stimulant-related Disorder*, etc.). *Tobacco-related Disorder* has also been added to the list of substances of abuse. Within each *Substance-related Disorder* exists a spectrum of severity described as *mild, moderate,* or *severe*. The severity is determined by the number of criteria a person meets. Each substance of abuse can be further delineated by whether the person is *intoxicated* or in *withdrawal*.

73

SUBSTANCE ABUSE AS A SPECTRUM OF ILLNESS

Another of the *8 Primary Spectrums of Mental Illness* is substance abuse. The global burden of substance abuse is enormous, and in the United States, the burden of tobacco, alcohol, and illicit drugs exceeds $600 billion annually.[29] In 2020, there were over 100,000 opioid overdose deaths. *Substance-related and Addictive Disorders* are a common primary diagnosis and are frequently a comorbid diagnosis. Clinicians cannot escape the importance of understanding substance abuse and its treatment. *Alcoholics Anonymous, Celebrate Recovery,* and other 12-step recovery groups are mainstays of treatment for many people. Treatment in the United States is delivered at different levels of care guided by the American Society of Addiction Medicine (ASAM) Criteria and include an array of options such as inpatient treatment, long-term residential treatment, outpatient programs, individual therapy, and medications. *Medication Assisted Treatment* (MAT) involves the use of methadone, Suboxone, naltrexone, Campral, and Antabuse for the treatment of *Opioid Use Disorder* and *Alcohol Use Disorder* with the first three of these interventions often being referred to as *Medication for Opioid Use Disorder* (MOUD). Nicotine replacement therapy, Chantix and Wellbutrin, as well as traditional psychiatric medication also have a role in treating *Substance Use Disorders*.

Certain ideas and words arising from the domain of addiction and its treatment have found their way into our lexicon. It is common to hear about various "addictions" like *sexual addictions, shopping addictions, nicotine addictions, caffeine addictions, workaholism, and Internet addictions*. Two of these involve a psychoactive compound that affects central nervous system receptors. The others rely upon the common denominator of *cravings* that addictive phenomena share. Many other words such as *codependency, dysfunctional, denial* and *dry drunk* have entered common usage. By extending the principles from the realm of addiction and recovery, we see that virtually any activity that brings pleasure and involves intense craving can be misused in an addictive manner.

When viewed through the lens of pleasure-seeking behavior and immediate gratification, *Substance-related and Addictive Disorders* share a great deal in common, regardless of the substance or behavior involved. There is a spectrum ranging from the ascetic to the person who chronically yields to pleasure-seeking and cravings. The middle region of this spectrum is epitomized by the adage *All things in moderation*. The caricatures depicted in the cartoons at the extreme are an "ascetic monk" and a "party animal" with raging addictions. In Analytical (Jungian) psychology, disavowing a psychic element and relegating it to the shadow, increases the likelihood of being overtaken or blindsided by it. We recall examples of evangelists and politicians who publicly rebuke sexual immorality only to be caught in the very same acts they denounce. From a Jungian perspective, the middle region of this spectrum is achieved via the *transcendent function* that fosters a *conjunctio*, or conjunction of opposites.

Ascetic Monk vs. Multiple Addictions:
"How Much PLEASURE Do You Seek?"

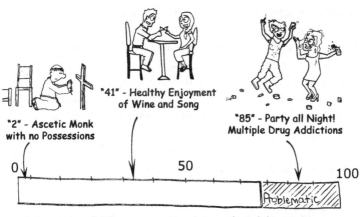

Amount of Pleasure Seeking / Addictiveness

St. Augstine
Madame Bovary constrained

St. Augstine the youth
Madame Bovary in passion

The spectrum of *Substance-Related and Addictive Disorder* is titled "Ascetic Monk vs. Multiple Addictions: How Much Pleasure Do You Seek?" The feature that determines where a person is on the spectrum involves the intensity of the craving and the pull toward pleasure-seeking behavior that a person experiences. Another way of looking at the spectrum is whether a person is overregulating his or her pleasure-seeking behavior versus overindulging those desires.

On the left side of the scale, the ascetic monk either lacks motivation and desire for pleasure or has so thoroughly restrained himself that the flames of passions are nearly extinguished. Such an ascetic lives simply, perhaps with few belongings. He is careful not to allow excessive excitement to inflame him. Such a person may be virtually celibate, austere, obedient, and abide by spartan rules. The material world and its pleasures do not hold sway in the person's life. Such a lifestyle befits an actual monk, but otherwise, it typically presents a problem. If such individuals seek treatment at all, they may need to surrender to pleasures and delights, loosen up, and have fun. Such persons seem incapable of enjoyment, not because they are depressed, but rather because pleasure-seeking is too tightly governed.

Consider, Maria, the novitiate in *The Sound of Music*. Her natural, irrepressibly joyful temperament was constrained by the monastic life. In fact, once Maria deals with her own excessive asceticism by becoming the children's nanny, she takes on the project of dismantling Captain von Trapp's regimented, overregulated household. The movie is an example of the tension between asceticism and indulgence. When love springs forth and Maria is confronted by the Mother Superior, she realizes that she has been hiding in the convent. She and Captain von Trapp are free to explore the vast middle region where pleasure dwells, but not to such excess that it enslaves them.

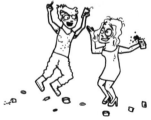

On the far right of the spectrum are people who might be described as "party animals." These people are almost entirely motivated by seeking pleasure. They rarely deny themselves anything. Rather, they are always reaching for the next thrill or another exciting experience. The ordinary life can be painful or distressing to them, so they often take risks to feel excitement, pleasure, and relief. The relief they seek leads to hazards, and such people are at high risk for addiction, often multiple addictions. They may get one addiction under control only to have another one spring up. In their thirst for pleasure and relief from distress, such people may become dependent on alcohol, pain medications, drugs of abuse (fentanyl, heroin, methamphetamine, etc), pornography, sex, tobacco, shopping, and a nearly endless list of other things associated with craving for pleasure that alleviates pain and discomfort. Denial is an integral part of substance use disorders, and sufferers seldom acknowledge that they have a problem. Eventually, when their *house of cards* collapses as a consequence of their addictions, they may be driven into some form of treatment. A partner may grow weary and become fed up, or a series of job losses, or infractions of the law occur before a person begins to face the reality of their substance use disorder. A popular idea in 12-Step Recovery circles is that a person must "hit rock bottom" before they are likely to admit they are powerless and that their life has become unmanageable. Only then does the long road to recovery begin in earnest. Treatment often includes participation in a 12-Step Recovery group or similar peer-led groups, individual therapy, and various levels of care from outpatient to inpatient and lots in between. Medications are used judiciously in people with addictions. Research concerning addiction offers promising possibilities for future treatments.[30] An enormously popular TED Talk by Johann Hari proposes that the opposite of addiction is human connection and many successful interventions like 12-Step Recovery can be understood as pathways toward restoring a person with substance use disorder into community.

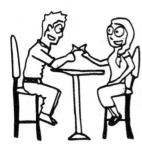

Like with all other *Spectrums of Mental Illness,* the optimal place to be on the scale of pleasure-seeking behavior is toward the middle. In that region, life is enjoyed, pleasure is sought, and the material world can be appreciated but without adverse consequences. Occasional splurges and moments of decadence are neither entirely absent nor do they dominate the background rhythm of a person's life. An occasional drink or a glass of wine may be consumed without problems ensuing. People with a propensity for addiction or who have family members with substance use disorders should exercise extra caution. In the middle part of the spectrum, people may drink responsibly; they recognize risks and can avoid them.

Present moment awareness is known to provide many benefits. Whether we choose to refer to this as *mindfulness, The Power of Now, carpe diem (seize the day), radical acceptance, practicing presence, contemplative living,* or *serenity,* these approaches share in common a surrender to living in the moment or *one day at a time.* For people with substance use disorder, these mindfulness-based strategies can provide a rich, vibrant way of living without the destructive patterns that occurred from their substance use.

CONCLUSION

A shift toward person-centered language that replaces *addict* with *person with a substance use disorder* or *clean time* with *substance-free period* seeks to reduce stigma; however, some of these terms still have their place.[31] The authors have occasionally used the term addiction while endorsing the shift toward more person-centered language. We cannot ignore that the etymology of addict refers to a person who has been bound over in servitude to a creditor. Insofar as a person with a substance use disorder becomes enslaved to the drug, the term addict has its place.

Sadly, *Substance-related and Addictive Disorders* are common. Addiction does not respect any ethnic, sociocultural, religious, racial, or other boundaries. These disorders are often recalcitrant, and treatment may be followed by relapse several times before sustained success is achieved. In 12-Step recovery groups, there exists a belief that untreated addiction inevitably leads to death or incarceration. Too often, that proves true. DSM-IV relied on a formulaic approach, where diagnosis depended on whether a person met criteria for the disorder. With the arrival of DSM-5 and DSM-5-TR, the clinician is encouraged to approach

Substance-related and Addictive Disorders as phenomena that exist along a spectrum. In addition, the particular substance of use appears less central to conceptualizing these disorders than the shared features of craving, high risk tolerance, and social impairment. On the *spectrum* presented in this chapter, each of us falls somewhere between the person cut off from all sensual pleasures and the person whose insatiable cravings rule his or her life.

CHAPTER 12

THE AUTISM SPECTRUM: CODEPENDENT VS. AUTISTIC

AUTISM—WHAT'S NEW IN DSM-5 & DSM-5-TR

DSM-5 gathered *Autism, Asperger's, Childhood Disintegrative Disorder* and *Pervasive Developmental Disorder NOS* into one diagnostic category known as *Autism Spectrum Disorder (ASD)*. Along with other diagnoses often presenting in childhood, *ASDs* are grouped under the broad heading of *Neurodevelopmental Disorders*. Considerable controversy and fear were stirred by the changes introduced with DSM-5 and perpetuated in DSM-5-TR. For instance, *Asperger's Syndrome*, a diagnosis that may have carried less stigma than *Autism*, is now subsumed by a diagnosis using the term *Autism*. *Autism Spectrum Disorder (ASD)* is characterized by 1) deficits in social communication and social interaction and 2) restricted repetitive behaviors. If only social communication and interaction are impaired, then *Social Communication Disorder* is diagnosed.

AUTISM AS A SPECTRUM OF ILLNESS

Added to the fact that *ASD* uses the word *spectrum* in its name, the popularization of *Asperger's Syndrome* contributed to the decision to include Autism as one of the *8 Primary Spectrums of Mental Illness*. When a diagnosis enters the lexicon to such an extent that *Asperger's* is tossed about as an adjective, it suggests the concept has captured something that was widely understood if not previously named. To say someone is *Asperger's* is frequently not synonymous with a formal diagnosis. Instead, it may imply that the subject's social skills are askew and that his or her capacity to interpret the social cues that most of us take for granted is impaired. Ironically, just as the concept of a spectrum of *Autism* and *Asperger's* has found its way into common usage, the DSM-5 removed *Asperger's* as a diagnosis. Concern has erupted over whether these changes will restrict or expand eligibility for services for children with ASD. However, a brief report in 2015 found that the label used had no bearing on the likelihood of harboring stereotypes, prejudice, or discriminatory attitudes.[32]

The scale used to illustrate this *Primary Spectrum of Mental Illness* depends upon an assessment of the degree to which a person is interpersonally connected, or "how connected to others are you?" This spectrum spans from individuals who are too connected to those who are almost completely unconnected. The choice of *un*-connected instead of *dis*-connected, reflects an appreciation for the fact that to become disconnected, one must first connect. Individuals with *ASD* typically struggle to connect in the first place.

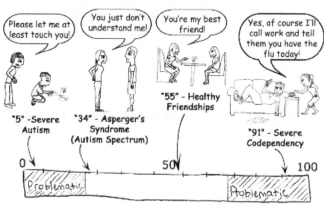

**Autism vs. Codependency:
How CONNECTED to Others are you?**

Degree of Connectedness to Others

THE AUTISM SPECTRUM: CODEPENDENT VS. AUTISTIC   83

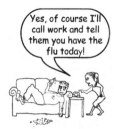

On the far-right end of the spectrum appear people who seem overly connected to others. They are people who become *enmeshed* and whose boundaries are too porous when it comes to the emotional lives of people around them. The term *Codependency* is used for the spectrum, though strictly speaking, it is a misapplication of the term. *Codependency* within the recovery movement pertains to the patterns in relationship wherein a person becomes "addicted" to managing the unmanageable behavior and consequences of their addicted partner. Whereas the addict is dependent upon a substance, the *codependent* person becomes dependent upon managing the addict. Nevertheless, the spectrum proposed here borrows the term *Codependency* because it aptly fits the sort of excessive and unhealthy connection that is intended.

In addition to the *enmeshed, codependent* quality that individuals at the extreme right side of the scale display, they often cannot tolerate being alone. They are overinvolved in others' lives. They frequently "need to feel needed," and they have difficulty when people in their circle exert independence from them. This may present particular problems when their children start to separate and become more independent. The overly connected person may gravitate toward people who lack the ability to manage their own lives effectively and who lack self-governance. In this respect, the term *Codependence* captures the idea well.

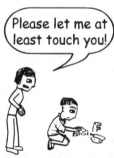

On the left end of the scale is the territory of *ASD*. The cartoon depicts the most extreme form of *Autism*, where even the most minimal interaction with others, like touch, can be experienced as disruptive. These people's difficulties in relationship began in early childhood; they did not relate like other children. Children with severe disorders often come to attention early and are seldom missed. They barely communicate, they engage in repetitive behaviors. Early intervention often includes intensive therapy, medication to manage behavior, and case management services. Diagnosis of children with less severe conditions may be delayed.

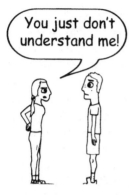

Further along toward the middle region, but still in a range where problems ensue, the person depicted would have been diagnosed with *Asperger's Syndrome* using DSM-IV criteria. The man's wife is exasperated by his utter lack of comprehension about the simplest sorts of things that most human beings understand. She is calling out to her husband, "You just don't understand me!" She is correct, because people with *Asperger's Syndrome* do not decipher ordinary social cues. When they do, it is often because they have learned a set of rules by rote memory that they apply in a stilted, predetermined fashion. Our character is a successful software engineer, in part, because he likes the logic that governs writing computer code. He trained to be an audiologist because the engineering and technology involved with testing equipment and amplification devices fascinated him but left that profession because he found the high demand for human interaction intolerable. He can still recite technical specifications for certain hearing aids from memory. His only friends were developed in high school, and they have always made allowances for him. Many people mistake his robotic manner for a lack of feeling and empathy, when in fact it is simply a feature of his poor ability to read social cues (his own and others).

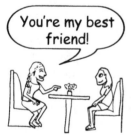

As always, the middle zone of this *spectrum* is the goal. Here we see two women enjoying lunch together. One exclaims that the other is her "best friend." There is a feeling of mutual friendship. Their care for one another is best described as *interdependent*. Individuals in the middle display the quality described by the Buddhist teacher Thich Nhat Hanh as *Inter-being*. This word, *Inter-being,* connotes a compassionate interconnectedness between all things. Such connectedness is vital, responsive, and meaningful, without the pitfalls of enmeshment, codependence, or overbearing control of other people.

CLINICAL EXAMPLE

Amanda was an oncology nurse whose life centered upon her only child. She presented for treatment two months after her son left for college. During her son's senior year of high school, she left her job doing direct patient care in hopes of enjoying more time at home with her son during his final year. Her husband worked in sales and drank excessively. Under the guise of wining and dining his clients, Amanda's husband tried to cover up his drinking. Amanda was endlessly picking up the slack for her husband. A month before their son left for college, her husband was charged with a DUI. He quit drinking and began attending AA meetings. Instead of late-night business meetings, he was now attending AA meetings every day of the week. When he would return from a meeting, he retired to his workshop, where he disappeared for hours at a time. As his involvement in AA continued, he began to really attend to the demands of his home life. This led Amanda to grow increasingly distressed, and she began to complain of feeling useless. She talked of feeling depressed and spoke of anxiety that she would end up all alone, with nobody to care for, no child, no husband, and no patients who needed her. For more than three months, she had not had to rush out of the house late at night to pick up her husband after receiving a call from a concerned client of his. It had also been three months since she made a call to her husband's employer to cover for him. She began to experience insomnia, crying spells, and pervasive anxiety. Amanda was on the far-right end of the scale where *codependency, enmeshed caretaking,* and *overly nurturing* behavior is rampant. She was prescribed an antidepressant, but more importantly, she entered therapy, where she dealt with her overly connected, enmeshed style of relating. She started attending *Al-Anon,* and the tools she acquired there proved invaluable in subduing a lifetime of codependent behavior.

CONCLUSION

This chapter presents a scale to illustrate one of the *8 Primary Spectrums of Mental Illness* based on the degree of connectedness a person displays. Along this scale from *Autism* to *Codependence* the pivotal question is "how connected are you?" Too much connectedness results in states of overenmeshment and codependency, where a person's ability to maintain appropriate boundaries is impaired. At the other extreme of connectedness, individuals are unable to connect with others or they are profoundly impaired in their ability to connect. The optimal region in the middle demonstrates a capacity for connection and interdependence that does not manifest in excessive connectedness or enmeshment.

CHAPTER 13

THE PERSONALITY SPECTRUM: NEUROTIC VS. OBNOXIOUS

PERSONALITY DISORDERS – WHAT'S NEW IN DSM-5/TR

The most drastic revision concerning personality disorders in DSM-5 and DSM-5-TR was the elimination of the multiaxial diagnostic system. The personality disorder diagnoses now appear like any other diagnosis. Though they remain grouped together, the personality disorder diagnoses were not eliminated. The criteria for personality disorders are nearly unchanged in DSM-5 and DSM-5-TR. *Antisocial Personality Disorder* also appears under the heading of *Disruptive, Impulse-Control, and Conduct Disorders*. This makes sense, as many clinicians observe that *Conduct Disorder* and *Oppositional Defiant Disorder* can be the predecessors of *Antisocial Personality Disorder*. All 10 personality disorders from DSM-IV were carried over into DSM-5 and DSM-5-TR.

PERSONALITY DISORDERS AS A SPECTRUM OF ILLNESS

The concept of personality fits very well into the conceptual framework of illness along a spectrum. The scale for personality disorders, another of the *8 Primary Spectrums of Mental Illness*, encompasses all 10 disorders. A fundamental feature of people with personality disorders is their tendency to *externalize* blame or causation for their symptoms.

Individuals with personality disorders have marked difficulty managing the daily affairs of their lives and their relationships with others. When something goes wrong, they immediately locate the source of their problems outside of themselves (this can also be described as having an *external locus of control*).[33] In contrast, the left side of the scale depicts individuals who would have been described as *neurotic* in DSM-II. At the extreme left end of the scale, the *neurotic* end, individuals ascribe to themselves exaggerated and excessive blame for anything that goes wrong.

People with personality disorders are also characterized by *rigidity* and *inflexibility* in the way they live and the way they relate to others. They have difficulty learning from experience and find it very difficult to change; they do not adapt. Repeated experiences that should demonstrate to the sufferer their role in their own struggles fail to inform them. Instead, when problematic patterns repeat, they simply reinforce their belief in an external cause and proceed to blame others. This is what is meant by *maladaptive*. Clinicians may find such patients' defenses to be almost impenetrable. It can be helpful to remember that people's inability to recognize their own role in the problems and the turmoil that surrounds them are pivotal features of personality disorders.

A certain amount of quirkiness and idiosyncrasy is to be expected across the range of normal human personality function. Looked at one way, everyone has certain personality traits that at one time or another are maladaptive and do not serve them well. However, personality disordered individuals display an exaggerated amount of idiosyncratic thought, perception, and behavior, and their difficulties are pervasive and persistent.

At either extreme of the scale outlined below, an individual is likely to have problems. Individuals located at the extreme left side of the scale locate the source of their problems within themselves. These are not people who know healthy guilt. Their guilt tends to be excessive and misappropriated. This excessive guilt can be erosive.

Healthy guilt can be distinguished from *neurotic* guilt by several features:

Healthy Guilt	vs	**Neurotic Guilt**
Arises from an act		Not easily associated with an act
Can be remedied or amended		No path to making things right
Yields better insight and living		Doomed to be repeated

The scale titled *Neurotic vs Obnoxious* highlights the polarity between blaming oneself too much and blaming others too much.

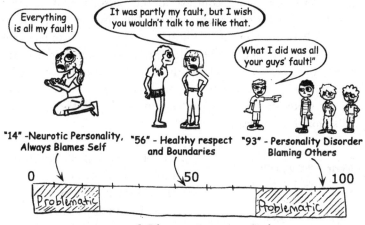

On the left end of the spectrum, *neurotic* individuals blame themselves too much and too often for things outside of their control. These people live in a state of perpetual anxiety that their blameworthiness will be revealed. Around every bend in life is some mishap or misfortune that is their fault or could be their fault. Their ability to fault themselves knows no bounds. They

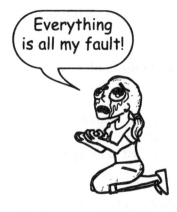

can easily recite the charges against themselves whether or not anyone asks them to do so. They may imagine wrongdoing where none occurred and reproach themselves or make exaggerated efforts to make amends. Woody Allen has made a career of portraying this sort of *neurotic* character in comical ways. His characters were racked with *neurotic* guilt and pervasive *anxiety*. While people at the extreme left end of the spectrum can prove frustrating and exhausting to their families and to clinicians trying to care for them, they often get along with others well enough since they are so appeasing. *Neurotic* individuals blame themselves but also endure the suffering that results. This is in stark contrast to the personality-disordered individual who not only blames others but also causes others to suffer with them. Certain medications offer limited relief from the associated anxiety. When their guilt and self-reproach are extreme or persistent, people on the *neurotic* end of the spectrum may be prescribed antidepressants, antianxiety agents, and sleeping medication to alleviate symptoms. Psychotherapy often yields more lasting results.

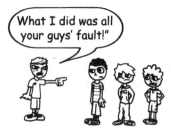

On the other end of the spectrum, the right side of the cartoon, is a figure depicting the personality-disordered domain. This person sees no fault in himself but sees endless fault in everyone else. Such individuals see the speck in the other person's eye while entirely missing the log in their own. The particular personality disorder chosen for the illustration was a young man with *Narcissistic Personality Disorder*, whose hubris leaves him feeling entitled to blame everyone but himself. People with other personality disorders like *Borderline Personality Disorder (BPD)* also tend to provoke very strong emotions in others, including clinicians. Clinicians must guard against acting upon the very intense, distorted projections that issue forth from the patient. This is sometimes terribly difficult to avoid since patients are adept at "stirring things up." Medications are rarely helpful; however, when symptoms of distressing emotions become severe enough, antidepressants, antianxiety agents, mood-stabilizing agents, antipsychotic agents, and sleeping agents are frequently employed. Though psychotherapy can be quite helpful in most instances, individuals with *Borderline* and *Narcissistic Personality Disorder* have difficulty tolerating the intensity of such a one-on-one psychotherapy relationship. People with *Borderline Personality Disorder* often find *Dialectical Behavior Therapy (DBT)* helpful, since this highly structured approach tends to diffuse some of the intensity of individual therapy while providing patients tools for regulating emotions and improving interpersonal effectiveness.

A recurrent problem in treating any of the personality disorders is their unyielding tendency to locate their difficulties outside themselves. Other people often recognize the need for treatment long before the sufferer does. Clinicians should remain alert for signs that the patient is distorting the relationship or blaming the clinician for their own behavior. After all, this feature is so entrenched that it rarely yields to life experience.

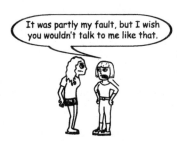

In the middle region, a person demonstrates the ability to accept responsibility for her actions, without unnecessary or exaggerated self-reproach. At the same time, a person in the middle is also able to discern that others sometimes share in responsibility and can be held accountable when something goes awry. In the middle of the *spectrum*, people demonstrate fluidity and flexibility in the way they adapt to challenges and problems that life presents. Holding the center of this *Spectrum* is particularly difficult, and too often the extremes are reserved for the ones closest to us.

CONCLUSION

Personality refers to those traits that are stable and persist over time. *Personality Disorders* are defined by persistent traits that are *maladaptive*. The central idea presented in this chapter is that *Personality Disorders* locate the cause of their problems outside themselves. This one trait makes it difficult to adapt to life's demands, since a person's efforts are directed almost exclusively to fixing others and not themselves. The *neurotic* end of the spectrum revolves around blaming oneself excessively. Here the impediment to change is the grip of unfounded self-reproach that tends to be self-defeating.

Life demands of each of us a willingness to accept our responsibility in matters that go wrong without yielding to an exaggerated degree of self- reproach or self-criticism. When that balance is struck, people learn from their mistakes, they cultivate a forgiving attitude toward themselves and others, and they develop the capacity to deal with the role they and others play in their misfortunes.

SECTION III
THE SECONDARY AREAS OF DIAGNOSIS

CHAPTER 14

THE SPECIALTY AREAS: (TRAUMA, NEURODEVELOPMENTAL, NEUROCOGNITIVE, BEHAVIORAL, DISSOCIATIVE, SOMATIC, EATING, ELIMINATION, SLEEP, SEXUAL, GENDER, PARAPHILIA)

The remaining sections of DSM-5-TR are covered in this chapter, titled *The Specialty Areas*. These disorders do not lend themselves as readily to inclusion as *Primary Spectrums*. To some degree, everyone has features associated with the *8 Primary Spectrums of Mental Illness*. The same cannot be said of the *The Specialty Areas*. Therefore, they are not depicted among the *Primary Spectrums of Mental Illness*. In time, Trauma- and Stress- Related Disorders may be reconceptualized as existing along a spectrum.

TRAUMA- AND STRESSOR-RELATED DISORDERS

Trauma- and Stressor-Related Disorders are very common. In a telephone interview study by Resnick, "Lifetime exposure to any type of significant traumatic event was 69%, whereas exposure to crimes that included sexual or aggravated assault or homicide of a close relative or friend occurred among 36%. Overall sample prevalence of *Posttraumatic Stress Disorder (PTSD)* was 12.3% lifetime and 4.6% within the past 6 months."[34] Individuals differ with regard to the effects they suffer when confronting a trauma or stress.

By segregating *Trauma- and Stressor-Related Disorders*, DSM-5-TR gives clear emphasis to "persistent negative alterations in mood and cognition." *Trauma- and Stressor-Related Disorders* include *Posttraumatic Stress Disorder (PTSD), Acute Stress Disorder, Adjustment Disorders,* and *Reactive Attachment Disorder.* In DSM-5-TR as with DSM-5, *PTSD* can be applied to individuals who experience trauma indirectly. Two subtypes are recognized, *Preschool Subtype* (<6 y.o.) and *Dissociative Subtype*. In DSM-5-TR *Adjustment Disorders* are recognized to be related to a stress and therefore have moved from the mood disorders section.

NEURODEVELOPMENTAL DISORDERS

The *Neurodevelopmental Disorders* include diagnoses that are typically recognized in childhood: *Autism Spectrum Disorder (ASD), Attention Deficit Hyperactivity Disorder (ADHD), Communication Disorder, Specific Learning Disorder,* and *Motor Disorders.*

ADHD is virtually unchanged. *Reading Disorder, Mathematics Disorder,* and *Disorder of Written Expression* have all been combined into *Specific Learning Disorder,* starting with DSM-5.

The diagnosis of *Mental Retardation* was replaced by *Intellectual Developmental Disorder.* This disorder is now assessed more by adaptive functioning and less by absolute IQ score.

NEUROCOGNITIVE DISORDERS

DSM-IV's diagnosis of *Dementia* saw a substantial shift in the new schema. The term *Dementia* was replaced with *Neurocognitive Disorder.* A spectrum of functioning is now recognized by distinguishing *Mild Neurocognitive Disorders* from *Major Neurocognitive Disorders.* The *Neurocognitive Disorders* include a long list of subtypes that specify the particular cause of the disorder. Subtypes include *Alzheimer's, Vascular, Substance Induced,*

Traumatic Brain Injury, HIV Infection, Parkinson's Disease, Lewy Bodies, Prion Disease, and Huntington's Disease.

DISRUPTIVE, IMPULSE-CONTROL, AND CONDUCT DISORDERS

Listed under this heading are *Oppositional Defiant Disorder, Conduct Disorder, Antisocial Personality Disorder, Pyromania, Kleptomania.*

DISSOCIATIVE DISORDERS

Dissociative Disorders comprises a separate category in DSM-5-TR, and *Depersonalization Disorder* was changed to *Depersonalization/ Derealization Disorder.* Dissociative Fugue is noted as a *Specifier* in DSM-5-TR.

SOMATIC DISORDERS

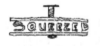

Somatic Symptom Disorder became a new construct starting with DSM-5. This disorder can easily be conceived as existing along a *spectrum* ranging from the previously recognized diagnosis of *Hypochondriasis* to *Somatization Disorder.* In DSM-5, *Somatization Disorder, Hypochondriasis, Pain Disorder,* and *Undifferentiated Somatoform Disorder* were all eliminated and replaced by the *Somatic Symptom Disorder Diagnosis.* The centerpiece of this disorder involves the extent to which the patient experiences distressing feelings, thoughts, or behaviors out of proportion to what might be expected from a condition. This disorder shifts the focus away from "unexplained medical symptoms." Clinicians may have experienced patients who were enraged by the implication that they had "made up" their symptoms. The introduction of *Somatic Symptom Disorder* helps to circumvent this issue.

In DSM-5-TR, *Conversion Disorder* was changed to *Functional Neurological Symptom Disorder.*

FEEDING AND EATING DISORDERS

 DSM-5 added a new category, *Feeding and Eating Disorders*, that is unchanged in DSM-5-TR. It encompasses eating disorders typically found in children, adolescents, and adults. *Pica* and *Rumination Disorder* can now be diagnosed at any age.

 Avoidant/Restrictive Food Intake Disorder is primarily intended to be used for children with extreme food preferences leading to substantial psychological or nutritional problems.

 Binge-Eating Disorder is for individuals who have weekly loss of control resulting in overeating leading to significant distress.

SLEEP DISORDERS

Starting with DSM-5, *Sleep Disorders* were recategorized to show a more fluid spectrum between medical and psychological issues. Primary insomnia was renamed *Insomnia Disorder*. Breathing-Related Sleep Disorders now include *Obstructive Sleep Apnea, Central Sleep Apnea,* and a category called *Sleep-Related Hypoventilation*.

 Rapid Eye Movement Sleep Behavior Disorder, and *Restless Leg Syndrome* were new for DSM-5.

GENDER DYSPHORIA

The introduction of *Gender Dysphoria* in DSM-5 represented an acknowledgment of the substantial psychological, political, and societal changes that had taken place during the past 30 years since the release of DSM-IV. The removal of the term *identity disorder* and its replacement with a concept of *gender incongruence,* which has the potential to produce *dysphoria,* may have lasting implications. To those in the LGBTQQIA+ (lesbian, gay, bisexual, transgendered, queer/questioning, intersex, asexual, and more) community, this new conceptualization gives more appropriate emphasis to the individuals' distress and dysphoria. By disengaging *Gender Dysphoria* from the category of sexual dysfunctions and paraphilias, where DSM-IV had placed it, the DSM-5 moved to decrease stigmatization.

DSM-5-TR made further refinements in the domain of gender issues with regard to nomenclature and in the relevant text. *Desired gender* was changed to *experienced gender. Cross-sex medical procedure* was changed to *gender-affirming medical procedure*; and *natal male/natal female* was changed to *individual assigned male/female at birth.*

SEXUAL DYSFUNCTIONS

The *Sexual Dysfunctions* section was reorganized in DSM-5. *Vaginismus* and *Dyspareunia* were removed from the manual and replaced with *Genito-Pelvic Pain/Penetration Disorder.* Furthermore, the diagnosis of *Sexual Aversion Disorder* was removed due to a lack of research evidence to support its inclusion.

PARAPHILIC DISORDERS

This category is virtually unchanged.

SECTION IV
CONCLUSIONS

CHAPTER 15

THE HARMONY OF THE LOTUS FLOWER

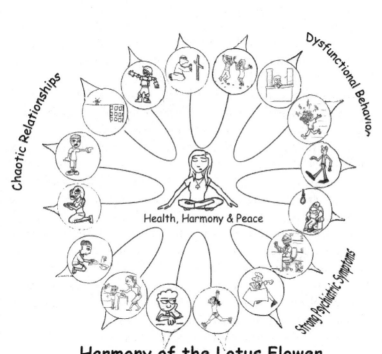

Harmony of the Lotus Flower

This mandala illustration summarizes our schema and points to a vision of how optimal functioning might look. It includes the *8 Primary Psychiatric Spectrums* radiating from the center of the lotus flower. The eight spectrums are paired and joined together with a curved line, whose apex comes together with the other pairs at the center of the flower. Thus, the portion comprising the apex of the curved line represents the middle range for each of the eight spectrums. This is the "sweet spot" that we try to attain for each continuum. On the periphery of the flower are the extreme ends of each spectrum. As there are eight primary psychiatric spectrums, there are 16 poles altogether, two for each spectrum. When we optimize each of the eight primary spectrums and find ourselves mostly in the center of the lotus, we achieve balance, flexibility, and adaptability. We represent this by the person peacefully meditating in the lotus flower's central space. Such states of balance may be elusive, but it is a personal call, a challenge.

This "center point" of the image is referred to by many names. It can be described as "being present in the moment," "living in the now," "staying aware," "being in flow," "being in the zone," "individuating," etc. This can be experienced as feeling closer to God or feeling intense clarity. As clinicians, our job is to assist clients in their struggles to pull toward the center of each of the eight spectrums and remain in that optimal zone.

The ultimate goal is to achieve a state where the dialectical splits of each spectrum are transcended. This involves holding the opposite ends of each spectrum in tension so that something new can emerge. The new state is more than a 50/50 balance between the opposite poles; it is entirely different. This centered, transcendent state preserves the best qualities of each extreme manifestation. We recognize this sort of transcendent function in figures like Martin Luther King Jr., Mahatma Gandhi, and Jesus. This conjunction of opposites fuels the process of individuation, whereby elements of the unconscious (personal and collective) become consciously integrated. To cultivate a life lived mostly in the center of the lotus is something akin to an ultimate call.

CHAPTER 16

CARL JUNG AND HIS RELATIONSHIP TO DSM-5-TR

The simplification of DSM-5-TR presented in this book fits well with most schools of psychology. It is equally at home with *Cognitive Behavioral Therapy, Object Relations, Self-Psychology, Emotion-Focused Therapy, Resilience Theory*, and other theoretical systems. Like the DSM, this book attempts to be "atheoretical," meaning it is much more descriptive and less representative of any particular theoretical perspective.

However, there is a decidedly *Jungian* aspect to the way this book presents the concept of *Spectrums of Illness*.

Carl Jung, a Swiss-born psychiatrist and contemporary of Sigmund Freud, was an original thinker and courageous explorer of the psyche. He and Freud parted ways in 1913, and Jung founded the *School of Analytical Psychology*. Some of the notable ideas introduced by Jung include *archetypes, collective unconscious, complexes, persona, shadow, introversion, extroversion*, and *individuation*.

Part of Jung's concept of the psyche includes a *transcendence of opposites*. Jung writes:

"The confrontation of the two positions generates a tension charged with energy and creates a living, third thing—not a logical stillbirth (...) but a movement out of the suspension between opposites, a living birth that leads to a new level of being, a new situation. The transcendent function manifests itself as a quality of conjoined opposites."
(Jung, CW 8, par. 189).

Elsewhere, he writes:

> "But if a union is to take place between opposites like spirit and matter, conscious and unconscious, bright and dark, and so on, it will happen in a third thing, which represents not a compromise but something new, just as for the alchemists the cosmic strife of the elements was composed by the stone that is no stone, by a transcendental entity that could be described only in paradoxes."
>
> (Jung, CW 14, par. 765)

Jung felt that one of the requirements of psychological growth was to learn how to hold polar opposites in tension within our psyche, despite their contradictions, and maintain that tension until a transcendent third element appeared. The transcendent third was not just a compromise between two opposites, but something entirely new, perhaps even revolutionary.

In our model, holding the opposites of the *8 Primary Psychiatric Spectrums* is not merely an attempt to stay in some sort of homeostatic balance. Ideally, it fosters the transcendence of opposites wherein a new state of consciousness and being can emerge. This is quite similar to Jung's description of the *transcendent function*. When this has been cultivated to a high degree, a person is free to be fully responsive to each moment. We are called to live as something bigger than the sum of our balanced parts. We are ultimately a transcendent spiritual being listening to a higher call. That is the ultimate *Harmony of the Lotus Flower*.

APPENDIX

ON ICD-10 AND THE DSM-5-TR

The *International Classification of Disease-10th Edition* (ICD-10) differs substantially from the DSM-5-TR. DSM-5-TR was developed by the *American Psychiatric Association* in order to better define clinical practice within mental health; it strives for a common diagnostic language. DSM- 5-TR's principal focus is improved clinical care through more accurate and widely accepted diagnoses. Practically, it is also a means by which insurance claims are coded and submitted for the purpose of reimbursement. ICD-10, on the other hand, is an international classification system developed by the *World Health Organization (WHO)* to provide uniform diagnoses in all fields of medicine worldwide. The greater specificity provided by ICD-10 diagnoses is expected to provide better information for identifying diagnosis, public health trends, epidemics, and even bioterrorism events. There is also a hope that precision in coding will result in fewer rejected claims, improved quality of care, and more useful benchmarks for data collection and analysis.

ICD-10's predecessor, ICD-9, had been in use in the United States for 35 years. ICD-9 had approximately 13,000 diagnostic codes; whereas, ICD-10 increased to a staggering 68,000 codes. ICD-10 went into effect in 2015.

ICD-10 substantially expanded how clinicians code their diagnoses for reimbursement. While ICD-9 had three to five digits per code, ICD-10 has up to seven digits per code. Many medical practitioners using ICD-10 must code each illness not only to a specific diagnosis but also a particular etiology, severity, and body location. This greatly adds to the length of the code and a multiplicity of variations to any category of diagnosis.

ICD-10 is divided into 26 sections, one for each letter of the alphabet. Thus, the 26 sections begin with A, B, C, D, etc. Each lettered section pertains to a different area of medicine. Sections A and B cover infectious diseases; section C is oncology; section D is hematology; and so on. The mental health codes appear in section F. Thus, virtually all the mental health codes begin with the letter F.

ICD-10's "F Section" for mental illness is broken down into 10 subsections as follows:

F01-F09 Mental disorders due to clear physiological conditions
F10-F19 Mental disorders due to substance abuse
F20-F29 Schizophrenia, schizotypal, delusional, and other psychotic processes F30-F39 Mood disorders
F40-F48 Anxiety, dissociative, stressor-related, and somatoform disorders F50-F59 Behavioral syndromes with physical factors
F60-F69 Personality disorder F70-F79 Intellectual disabilities
F80-F89 Pervasive developmental disorders
F90-F98 Disorders of childhood and adolescence F99-F99 Unspecified mental disorders

This book includes a front section with the majority of DSM-5-TR as well as ICD-10 summarized into a few pages. This is meant to serve as a quick reference for the commonly diagnosed mental disorders. While it summarizes the diagnostic criterion, it does not have the entire set of criteria. Reviewing these pages will give you a quick refresher of both systems.

ENDNOTES

[1] Kapur, S., A. G. Phillips, and T. R. Insel. "Why Has It Taken so Long for Biological Psychiatry to Develop Clinical Tests and What to Do about It?" *Molecular Psychiatry* 17, no. 12 (2012): 1174-179.

[2] Insel, Thomas. "Director's Blog: Transforming Diagnosis." NIMH RSS. April 29, 2013. Accessed September 14, 2014. http://www.nimh.nih.gov/about/director/2013/transforming-diagnosis.shtml.

[3] Jung, C. G. "The Phenomenology of the Spirit in Fairytales." In *Collected Works of C.G. Jung Volume 9, Part 1: The Archetypes and the Collective Unconscious*, 426. Vol. 9. London: Routledge and Kegan Paul, 1959.

[4] Jung, C. G. "The Phenomenology of the Spirit in Fairytales." In *Collected Works of C.G. Jung Volume 9, Part 1: The Archetypes and the Collective Unconscious*, 397. Vol. 9. London: Routledge and Kegan Paul, 1959.

[5] "And do not give the weak-minded your property, which Allah has made a means of sustenance for you, but provide for them with it and clothe them and speak to them words of appropriate kindness." "Surat An-Nisā' (The Women)" -Surat An-Nisa' [4:5]. Accessed September 14, 2014. http://quran.com/4/5.

[6] Hart, Rachel. "(N)either Men (n)or Women: The Failure of the Western Binary System", retrieved on February 5, 2022 at https://classicalstudies.org/annual-meeting/148/abstract/neither-men-nor-women-failure-western-binary-systems.

[7] Styron, William. *"Darkness Visible: A Memoir of Madness.* New York, NY. Vintage Books. 1992.

[8] *Diagnostic and Statistical Manual of Mental Disorders: DSM-5.* Washington, D.C.: American Psychiatric Association, 2013. 271

[9] Ryman, F. V. M., Cesuroglu, T., Bood, Z. M., and Syurina E.V. (2019) Orthorexia Nervosa: Disorder or Not? Opinions of Dutch Health Professionals. *Front. Psychol.* 10:555. doi: 10.3389/fpsyg.2019.00555.

[10] Bento, B. The review process of the DSM 5: is gender a cultural or diagnostic category?. Sociol Int J. 2018;2(3):205-213.

[11] Carotenuto, Aldo. *The Difficult Art.* Asheville NC, Chiron Publications, 2013.

[12] Angst, J. "The Bipolar Spectrum." *The British Journal of Psychiatry* 190, no. 3 (2007): 189-91.

[13] Hollingworth, Leta Stetter. *Functional Periodicity; an Experimental Study of the Mental and Motor Abilities of Women during Menstruation.* New York: Teachers College, Columbia University, 1914.

[14] Bell, Susan E., and Susan M. Reverby. "Vaginal Politics: Tensions and Possibilities in The Vagina Monologues." *Women's Studies International Forum* 28, no. 5 (2005): 430-44.

[15] Studd, J. (2012). Severe premenstrual syndrome and bipolar disorder: a tragic confusion. *Menopause International, 18*(2), 82–86.

[16] Greenberg, P.E., Fournier, A.A., Sisitsky, T. *et al.* The Economic Burden of Adults with Major Depressive Disorder in the United States (2010 and 2018). *PharmacoEconomics* **39,** 653–665 (2021).

[17] Angst, J., Gamma, A., Clarke, D., Ajdacic-Gross, V., Rossler, W., and Regier, D. "Subjective Distress Predicts Treatment Seeking for Depression, Bipolar, Anxiety, Panic, Neurasthenia and Insomnia Severity Spectra." *Acta Psychiatrica Scandinavica* 122, no. 6 (2010): 488-98.

[18] Angst, J. "Bipolar Disorders in DSM-5: Strengths, Problems and Perspectives." *International Journal of Bipolar Disorders* 1, no. 1 (2013): 12.

[19] Moreno, C., Laje, G., Blanco, C., Jiang, H., Schmidt, A. B., and Olfson, M. "National Trends in the Outpatient Diagnosis and Treatment of Bipolar Disorder in Youth." *Archives of General Psychiatry* 64, no. 9 (2007): 1032-039.

[20] Sadock, V. A. "Anxiety Disorders." In *Kaplan & Sadock's Concise Textbook of Clinical Psychiatry,* by Benjamin Jesse Saddock. 3rd ed. Philadelphia, PA: Lippincott Williams & Wilkins, 2012.

ENDNOTES

[21] Silberman, E., Balon, R., Starcevic, V., Shader, R., Cosci, F., Fava, G., Sonino, N. (2021). Benzodiazepines: It's time to return to the evidence. The *British Journal of Psychiatry, 218(3), 125-127.*

[22] Stein, D. J., Lim, C. C. W., Roest, A. M., de Jonge, .P, et al, WHO World Mental Health Survey Collaborators BMC Med. 2017; 15(1): 143.

[23] Jakubietz, M., Jakubietz, R. J., Kloss, D. F., and Gruenert, J. J. "Body Dysmorphic Disorder: Diagnosis and Approach." *Plastic and Reconstructive Surgery* 119, no. 6 (2007): 1924-930.

[24] Gittelman, R., Mannuzza, S. Shenker, R., and Bonagura, N. "Hyperactive Boys Almost Grown Up: I. Psychiatric Status." *Archives of General Psychiatry* 42, no. 10 (1985): 937-47.

[25] Mannuzza, S., R. G. Klein, N. Bonagura, P. H. Konig, and R. Shenker. "Hyperactive Boys Almost Grown Up: II. Status of Subjects Without a Mental Disorder." *Archives of General Psychiatry* 45, no. 1 (1988): 13-18.

[26] Mannuzza, S., Klein, R. G., Konig, P. H., and Giampino, T. L. "Hyperactive Boys Almost Grown Up: IV. Criminality and Its Relationship to Psychiatric Status." *Archives of General Psychiatry* 46, no. 12 (1989): 1073–079.

[27] Mannuzza, S., Klein, R. G., Bonagura, N., Malloy, P., Giampino, T. L., and Addalli, K. A. "Hyperactive Boys Almost Grown Up: V. Replication of Psychiatric Status." *Archives of General Psychiatry* 48, no. 1 (1991): 77–83. doi:10.1001/archpsyc.1991.01810250079012.

[28] Group, The Mta Cooperative. "A 14-Month Randomized Clinical Trial of Treatment Strategies for Attention-Deficit/Hyperactivity Disorder." *Archives of General Psychiatry* 56, no. 12 (1999):1073–086.

[29] Rehm, J., Mathers, C., Popova, S., Thavorncharoensap, M. Teerawattananon, Y., and Patra, J. "Global Burden of Disease and Injury and Economic Cost Attributable to Alcohol Use and Alcohol-use Disorders." *The Lancet* 373, no. 9682 (2009): 2223–233.

[30] Sanjakdar, S. S., Madoon, P. P., Marks, M. J., Bruznell, D. H., Maskos, U., McIntosh, M. Bowers, S. and Damaj, I. "Differential Roles of $\alpha 6\beta 2$ and $\alpha 4\beta 2$ Neuronal Nicotinic Receptors in Nicotine- and Cocaine-Conditioned Reward in Mice." *Neuropsychopharmacology*, July 18, 2014. Accessed October 3, 2014.

[31] Fisher, C. E. *The Urge: Our History of Addiction.* Penguin Press, New York, NY, 2022.

[32] Ohan, J.L., Ellefson, S.E., Corrigan, P.W. Brief Report: The Impact of Changing from DSM-IV 'Asperger's' to DSM-5 'Autistic Spectrum Disorder' Diagnostic Labels on Stigma and Treatment Attitudes. *J Autism Dev Disord* **45,** 3384–3389 (2015).

[33] Rotter, J. B. "Generalized Expectancies for Internal versus External Control of Reinforcement." *Psychological Monographs: General and Applied* 80, no. 1 (1966): 1–28.

[34] Resnick, H. S., Kilpatrick, D. G., Dansky, B. S., Saunders, B. E., et. al. "Prevalence of Civilian Trauma and Post Traumatic Stress Disorder in a Representative National Sample of Women." *Journal of Consulting and Clinical Psychology* 61, no. 6 (1993): 984–91.

INDEX

A
Addiction xv, 73, 74, 77, 78, 111
Agoraphobia xiii, 11, 53, 47
American Psychiatric Association 11, 99, 113
Antisocial Personality Disorder xxviii, 87, 97
Anxiety Disorders xiii, 20, 53, 57, 65, 110
Asperger's Syndrome 81, 84
Attention Deficit Hyperactivity Disorder (ADHD) 23, 65, 66, 71, 96, 111
Autism Spectrum Disorder (ASD) xvi, 16, 23, 29, 81, 96

B
Bipolar Disorders xi, 110
  Bipolar I Disorder xi
  Bipolar II Disorder xi
  Cyclothymic Disorder xi, 16
  Hypomanic Episode xi
Bipolarity 5, 6, 48, 50, 51,
Body Dysmorphic Disorder xiv, 21, 65, 70, 111
Breathing Related Sleep Disorders xxiv, 26, 98
  Central Sleep Apnea xxiv, 26, 98
  Obstructive Sleep Apnea Hypopnea xxiv
  Sleep-Related Hypoventilation xxiv, 26, 98

C
Conduct Disorder xxi, 87, 97

D
Delusional Disorder xii, 63
Depression xii, 19, 20, 21, 29, 31, 39, 44, 59, 110
Dialectical Behavior Therapy 91
Disruptive Impulse-Control Disorders xxi
Disruptive Mood Dysregulation Disorder x, 40
Dissociative Disorders xviii, 6, 25, 97
Dissociative Identity Disorder (Multiple Personality) DSM xviii

DSM-I 11
DSM-II 11, 12, 88
DSM-III 12–14, 19, 20, 26
DSM-III-R 12
DSM-IV 4, 5, 9, 13–15, 19, 20, 23, 26, 30, 41, 47, 84, 87, 98, 99, 112
DSM-IV-TR 13
Dysthymia x, 20, 39
Dysthymic Disorder 19, 20, 39, 44

E
Eating Disorders
  Anorexia Nervosa xix, 26
  Binge Eating Disorder xix, 26, 98
  Bulimia Nervosa xix, 26
Elimination Disorders xix, 6
Encopresis xix
Enuresis xix
Excoriation Disorder 21

F
Feeding Disorders xix

G
Gambling Disorder xv, 22, 73
Gender Dysphoria xxv, 6, 26, 27, 98
Generalized Anxiety Disorder xiii, 55

H
Hoarding Disorder xiv, 21, 65, 70

I
ICD-6 11
ICD-8 11
ICD-9 ix, 7, 12, 13, 107
ICD-10 ix, 7, 9, 13, 107, 108
International Classification of Disease. *See* ICD

L
Lotus Flower 6, 103, 106

M
Major Depressive Disorder ix, 16, 44, 57, 110
Mania 31, 47
Mental Retardation 12, 23, 96

N
Neurocognitive Disorders
  Delirium xx, 16
  Major Neurocognitive Disorder xx, 96
  Mild Neurocognitive Disorders xx, 96
Neurodevelopmental Disorders 23, 81, 96

O
Obsessive Compulsive Disorder xiv, 20, 65, 66, 69

P
Panic Disorder xiii, 55, 56
Paraphilic Disorders xxvi, 6
Parasomnias xxiv
Personality Disorders xxvii, 12, 92

Antisocial Personality
    Disorder xxviii, 87, 97
Avoidant Personality
    Disorder xxix
Borderline Personality
    Disorder xxviii, 90, 91
Dependent Personality
    Disorder xxix
Histrionic Personality
    Disorder xxviii
Narcissistic Personality
    Disorder xxviii, 90
Obsessive-Compulsive
    Personality Disorder xxix
Paranoid Personality
    Disorder xxvii
Schizoid Personality
    Disorder xxvii
Schizotypal Personality
    Disorder xxvii
Post Traumatic Stress Disorder
    (PTSD) xvii, 20, 24, 112
Premenstrual Dysphoric
    Disorder x, 20, 40, 45
Psychosis 31, 59, 63, 64
Psychotic Disorders xii

S

Schizoaffective Disorder xii, 63
Schizophrenia xii, 21, 59, 63, 108
Selective Mutism xiii, 17, 53
Separation Anxiety Disorder
    xiii, 53
Sexual Disorders xxv
Sleep Disorders xxiv, 26, 98
Somatic Disorders xxii
Somatic Symptom Disorder
    xxii, 25, 97
Substance Abuse xv, 21, 31, 73

T

Tobacco Use Disorder xv, 22
Transcendence of opposites 105
Transcendent function 75, 104, 105, 106
Trauma-Related Disorders 24
Trichotillomania xiv, 21, 65, 70

W

World Health Organization
    (WHO) 107

Made in the USA
Middletown, DE
01 November 2024